Update on Motion Preservation Technologies

Editor

DOMAGOJ CORIC

NEUROSURGERY CLINICS OF NORTH AMERICA

www.neurosurgery.theclinics.com

Consulting Editors
RUSSELL R. LONSER
DANIEL K. RESNICK

October 2021 • Volume 32 • Number 4

ELSEVIER

1600 John F. Kennedy Boulevard • Suite 1800 • Philadelphia, Pennsylvania, 19103-2899

http://www.theclinics.com

NEUROSURGERY CLINICS OF NORTH AMERICA Volume 32, Number 4
October 2021 ISSN 1042-3680, ISBN-13: 978-0-323-81054-8

Editor: Stacy Eastman
Developmental Editor: Ann Gielou Posedio

Photocopying

Single photocopies of single articles may be made for personal use as allowed by national copyright laws. Permission of the Publisher and payment of a fee is required for all other photocopying, including multiple or systematic copying, copying for advertising or promotional purposes, resale, and all forms of document delivery. Special rates are available for educational institutions that wish to make photocopies for non-profit educational classroom use. For information on how to seek permission visit www.elsevier.com/permissions or call: (+44) 1865 843830 (UK)/(+1) 215 239 3804 (USA).

Derivative Works

Subscribers may reproduce tables of contents or prepare lists of articles including abstracts for internal circulation within their institutions. Permission of the Publisher is required for resale or distribution outside the institution. Permission of the Publisher is required for all other derivative works, including compilations and translations (please consult www.elsevier.com/permissions).

Electronic Storage or Usage

Permission of the Publisher is required to store or use electronically any material contained in this periodical, including any article or part of an article (please consult www.elsevier.com/permissions). Except as outlined above, no part of this publication may be reproduced, stored in a retrieval system or transmitted in any form or by any means, electronic, mechanical, photocopying, recording or otherwise, without prior written permission of the Publisher.

Notice

No responsibility is assumed by the Publisher for any injury and/or damage to persons or property as a matter of products liability, negligence or otherwise, or from any use or operation of any methods, products, instructions or ideas contained in the material herein. Because of rapid advances in the medical sciences, in particular, independent verification of diagnoses and drug dosages should be made.

Although all advertising material is expected to conform to ethical (medical) standards, inclusion in this publication does not constitute a guarantee or endorsement of the quality or value of such product or of the claims made of it by its manufacturer.

Neurosurgery Clinics of North America (ISSN 1042-3680) is published quarterly by Elsevier Inc., 360 Park Avenue South, New York, NY 10010-1710. Months of issue are January, April, July, and October. Business and Editorial Offices: 1600 John F. Kennedy Blvd., Suite 1800, Philadelphia, PA 19103-2899. Customer Service Office: 11830 Westline Industrial Drive, St. Louis, MO 63146. Periodicals postage paid at New York, NY, and additional mailing offices. Subscription prices are $438.00 per year (US individuals), $1,013.00 per year (US institutions), $470.00 per year (Canadian individuals), $1,059.00 per year (Canadian institutions), $545.00 per year (international individuals), $1,059.00 per year (international institutions), $100.00 per year (US students), $255.00 per year (international students), and $100.00 per year (Canadian students). International air speed delivery is included in all *Clinics* subscription prices. All prices are subject to change without notice. **POSTMASTER:** Send address changes to *Neurosurgery Clinics of North America*, Elsevier Periodicals Customer Service, 11830 Westline Industrial Drive, St. Louis, MO 63146. **Customer Service: 1-800-654-2452 (US and Canada). From outside the US and Canada, call: 1-314-453-7041. Fax: 1-314-453-5170. E-mail: JournalsCustomerService-usa@elsevier.com (for print support) and journalsonlinesupport-usa@elsevier.com (for online support).**

Reprints. For copies of 100 or more, of articles in this publication, please contact the Commercial Reprints Department, Elsevier Inc., 360 Park Avenue South, New York, NY 10010-1710. Tel. 212-633-3874; Fax: 212-633-3820; E-mail: reprints@elsevier.com.

Neurosurgery Clinics of North America is covered in *MEDLINE/PubMed (Index Medicus), EMBASE/Excerpta Medica, and Current Contents/Clinical Medicine (CC/CM).*

Contributors

CONSULTING EDITORS

RUSSELL R. LONSER, MD
Professor and Chair, Department of
Neurological Surgery, The Ohio State
University Wexner Medical Center, Columbus,
Ohio, USA

DANIEL K. RESNICK, MD, MS
Professor and Vice Chairman, Program
Director, Department of Neurosurgery,
University of Wisconsin-Madison School of
Medicine and Public Health, Madison,
Wisconsin, USA

EDITOR

DOMAGOJ CORIC, MD
Professor, Department of Orthopedics, Spine
Division Chief, Atrium Healthcare
Musculoskeletal Institute, Carolina
Neurosurgery and Spine Associates, Charlotte,
North Carolina, USA

AUTHORS

KINGSLEY ABODE-IYAMAH, MD
Assistant Professor, Department of
Neurosurgery, Mayo Clinic, Jacksonville,
Florida, USA

TIM ADAMSON, MD
Carolina Neurosurgery and Spine Associates,
Atrium Health Musculoskeletal Institute,
Charlotte, North Carolina, USA

JOSEPH L. ALBANO, DO
Spine Surgery Fellow, Texas Back Institute,
Texas Back Institute, Plano, Texas, USA

ÓSCAR L. ALVES, MD
Head of Neurosurgery, Hospital Lusíadas
Porto, Senior Consultant in Neurosurgery,
Centro Hospitalar de Gaia/Espinho, Porto,
Portugal; Fulbright Fellow, CSRS-E Treasurer
and Executive Board member, WFNS Spine
Committee Board Member

MOHAMMED ALI ALVI, MBBS, MS
Postdoctoral Research Fellow, Mayo Clinic
Neuro-Informatics Laboratory, Department of
Neurologic Surgery, Department of

Neurosurgery, Mayo Clinic, Rochester,
Minnesota, USA

ANTHONY M. ASHER, BA
University of North Carolina School of
Medicine, Charlotte, North Carolina, USA

RACHEL BLUE, MD
Department of Neurosurgery, Perelman School
of Medicine, University of Pennsylvania,
Philadelphia, Pennsylvania, USA

MOHAMAD BYDON, MD
Professor of Neurosurgery, Orthopedics, and
Health Services Research, Mayo Clinic Neuro-
Informatics Laboratory, Department of
Neurologic Surgery, Department of
Neurosurgery, Mayo Clinic, Rochester,
Minnesota, USA

GREGORY CALLANAN, DO
Department of Orthopedic Surgery, Inspira
Health Network, Vineland, New Jersey, USA

DOMAGOJ CORIC, MD
Professor, Department of Orthopedics, Spine
Division Chief, Atrium Healthcare

Musculoskeletal Institute, Carolina Neurosurgery and Spine Associates, Charlotte, North Carolina, USA

DANIEL FRANCO, MD
Department of Neurological Surgery, Thomas Jefferson University Hospitals, Philadelphia, Pennsylvania, USA

GLENN A. GONZALEZ, MD
Department of Neurological Surgery, Thomas Jefferson University Hospitals, Philadelphia, Pennsylvania, USA

ANSHIT GOYAL, MBBS, MS
Postdoctoral Research Fellow, Mayo Clinic Neuro-Informatics Laboratory, Department of Neurologic Surgery, Department of Neurosurgery, Mayo Clinic, Rochester, Minnesota, USA

BEN JIAHE GU, MD
Department of Neurosurgery, Perelman School of Medicine, University of Pennsylvania, Philadelphia, Pennsylvania, USA

RICHARD D. GUYER, MD
Chairman, Texas Back Institute Research Foundation, Co-Director, Center for Disc Replacement at Texas Back Institute, Texas Back Institute, Plano, Texas, USA

JAMES HARROP, MD, MSHQS
Department of Neurological Surgery, Thomas Jefferson University Hospitals, Philadelphia, Pennsylvania, USA

ROBERT M. HAVEY, MS
Musculoskeletal Biomechanics Laboratory, Edward Hines, Jr. VA Hospital, Hines, Illinois, USA

KEVIN HINES, MD
Department of Neurological Surgery, Thomas Jefferson University Hospitals, Philadelphia, Pennsylvania, USA

GARRETT LARGOZA, BA
Department of Neurological Surgery, Thomas Jefferson University Hospitals, Philadelphia, Pennsylvania, USA

GIORGOS D. MICHALOPOULOS, MD
Postdoctoral Research Fellow, Mayo Clinic Neuro-Informatics Laboratory, Department of Neurologic Surgery, Department of

Neurosurgery, Mayo Clinic, Rochester, Minnesota, USA

THIAGO S. MONTENEGRO, MD
Department of Neurological Surgery, Thomas Jefferson University Hospitals, Philadelphia, Pennsylvania, USA

PIERCE NUNLEY, MD
Spine Institute of Louisiana, Shreveport, Louisiana, USA

DONNA D. OHNMEISS, PhD
President, Texas Back Institute Research Foundation, Texas Back Institute, Plano, Texas, USA

JONATHAN M. PARISH, MD
Department of Neurological Surgery, Carolinas Medical Center, Charlotte, North Carolina, USA

AVINASH G. PATWARDHAN, PhD
Director, Musculoskeletal Biomechanics Laboratory, Edward Hines, Jr. VA Hospital, Hines, Illinois, USA; Professor, Department of Orthopedic Surgery and Rehabilitation, Loyola University Medical Center, Maywood, Illinois, USA

RICHARD L. PRICE, MD, PhD
Complex and Minimally Invasive Spine Fellow, Department of Neurological Surgery, Washington University School of Medicine, St Louis, Missouri, USA; Swedish Neuroscience Institute, Seattle, Washington, USA

KRISTEN E. RADCLIFF, MD, FAAOS
Department of Orthopedic Surgery, Thomas Jefferson University, Rothman Institute, Egg Harbor Township, New Jersey, USA

WILSON Z. RAY, MD
Professor of Neurosurgery, Chief of Spine, Washington University School of Medicine, St Louis, Missouri, USA

VINCENT ROSSI, MD, MBA
Carolina Neurosurgery and Spine Associates, Atrium Health Musculoskeletal Institute, Charlotte, North Carolina, USA

KELLY (FRANK) VAN SCHOUWEN, MS
Spine Institute of Louisiana, Shreveport, Louisiana, USA

MARCUS STONE, PhD
Spine Institute of Louisiana, Shreveport,
Louisiana, USA

WILLIAM C. WELCH, MD, FACS, FICS
Department of Neurosurgery, Perelman School
of Medicine, University of Pennsylvania,
Philadelphia, Pennsylvania, USA

JANG YOON, MD
Department of Neurosurgery, Perelman School
of Medicine, University of Pennsylvania,
Philadelphia, Pennsylvania, USA

Contents

Cervical total disc replacement devices have been marketed in the United States (US) since 2007, with abundant level 1 evidence published on the treatment. Adherence to the strict inclusion/exclusion criteria and the surgical technique training of the US clinical trials remains the consistent and conservative approach to patient selection and implantation technique. However, patient selection and surgical technique remain debated among US surgeons as the published data and available cervical total disc replacements continue to grow.

The first US Food and Drug Administration (FDA) approval for cervical total disc replacement (CTDR) was issued in 2007. Since then, 8 more artificial discs have been granted FDA approval for single-level CTDR. Two of these have also been approved for 2-level CTDR. All devices are indicated for levels C3 to C7 for symptomatic patients with radiculopathy or myelopathy caused by disc herniation or spondylosis unresponsive to conservative management. Trials have shown noninferiority of CTDR compared with anterior cervical decompression and fusion in their overall success. Hybrid surgery and CTDR of 3 or more levels are not FDA approved.

Cervical total disc replacement (cTDR) is now a firm alternative to anterior cervical discectomy and fusion (ACDF) for degenerative disc disease (DDD). Robust level 1 data from Federal Drug Administration–approved clinical trials demonstrated that cTDR is in any case equally safe and effective compared with ACDF for 1- or 2-level DDD. Furthermore, from early postoperative to long-term follow-up of 10 to 15 years, cTDR rates superiorly in many primary clinical outcomes. According to the published literature, at least nine different cTDR devices share this consistent pattern. On the other hand, the surgical treatment of more than 2-level disc disease is haunted by an elusive paradox. It is easily understandable that 3- and 4-level ACDF, with the well-known associated limitations, is not the superlative intervention for a spine segment anatomically designed to provide motion, as cervical spine is. Furthermore, multilevel ACDF exacerbates many of the clinical and biomechanical complications related with single-level fusion. However, as cTDR is not immaculate of constraints and failures, its clinical safety and efficacy and cost-effectiveness in multilevel anterior compressive pathology need to be established. This article analyses the current available evidence supporting the expanded indication of cTDR to 3- and 4-level disc disease, either stand-alone or adjacent to fusion, from a less stringent European perspective.

Prosthesis design has an influence on the quantity and quality of postoperative motion after cervical disc arthroplasty. Prostheses with built-in resistance to angular and translational motion may have an advantage in restoring physiologic motion. The ability of a prosthesis to work with remaining bony and soft tissues to restore motion and load-sharing is a function of the kinematic degrees of freedom DOF, axis of rotation for a given motion, and device stiffness. How these characteristics allow the prosthesis to work with the patient's anatomy will determine whether the prosthesis is successful at restoring motion and mitigating adjacent-level stresses.

Intuitively, the introduction of artificial discs into spinal surgery offered the promise of reducing the incidence of adjacent segment (AS) reoperation compared with fusion. Several early clinical studies reported nonstatistically significant differences in AS disease between total disc replacement and fusion. Given the relatively low rate of AS reoperation ($\sim$1%–2% per year) following fusion, any appropriately powered study designed to demonstrate a statistically significant difference compared with arthroplasty would require thousands of patients and/or long-term follow-up (>5 years). Therefore, these differences only become apparent with large study size or meta-analyses and longer follow-up.

Low back pain is the leading cause of disability worldwide in industrialized nations. The pathology underlying chronic low back pain is associated with numerous factors. Lumbar degenerative disc disease is a potential major source of low back pain. There are numerous treatment modalities and options. Nonsurgical treatment options exist in the form of pain management through a combination of anti-inflammatory medications and steroid injections, physical therapy and lifestyle modifications. This article reviews the history and current trends in use for lumbar toral disc arthroplasty for degenerative disc disease treatment. Furthermore, indications, contraindications, and complications management are discussed.

There is an ongoing desire for the development of motion-preserving facet replacement devices as an alternative to rigid fixation in hopes of better preserving the natural kinematics of the lumbar spine. Theoretically, such a construct would simultaneously address pain associated with spinal instability and prevent abnormal load distribution and adjacent segment degeneration. Several such devices have been developed including the Anatomic Facet Replacement System, the Total Facet Arthroplasty System, and the Total Posterior Arthroplasty System. Of these devices, none have yet proven to be more efficacious than rigid fixation for lumbar spinal stenosis, and studies are ongoing.

NEUROSURGERY CLINICS OF NORTH AMERICA

SERIES OF RELATED INTEREST

Neurologic Clinics
https://www.neurologic.theclinics.com/
Neuroimaging Clinics
https://www.neuroimaging.theclinics.com/

THE CLINICS ARE AVAILABLE ONLINE!
Access your subscription at:
www.theclinics.com

Preface
Update on Spinal Arthroplasty

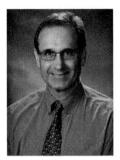

Domagoj Coric, MD
Editor

The majority of this Update on Motion Preservation Technologies is dedicated to cervical arthroplasty, owing to the quicker and more pervasive adoption of total disc replacement (TDR) devices in the cervical spine. The disparity in acceptance of this novel technology is multifactorial, but lies largely in the familiarity of the anterior cervical approach to spine surgeons as well as the straightforward nature of the diagnosis of cervical radiculopathy. Conversely, the anterior lumbar approach is more precarious, generally requiring an exposure surgeon, and the surgical treatment of mechanical low-back pain remains somewhat controversial. Some innovative devices are poised to bring arthroplasty to the lumbar spine from a posterior approach in the near future.

Rudimentary attempts at spine arthroplasty date back to the 1960s.[1] The modern era of spinal arthroplasty began with the introduction of the SB Charite I Artificial Disc in the lumbar spine (developed in 1982 in Germany; Food and Drug Administration [FDA]-approved in 2004 as the SB Charite III)[2] and the Bristol-Cummings Disc in the cervical spine (developed in the 1990s in England; FDA-approved in 2006 as the Prestige ST).[3] This new era of spine arthroplasty was ushered in with equal parts fanfare and skepticism. What followed was an unprecedented burst of scientific inquiry producing an unparalleled volume of level I and II evidence comparing arthroplasty to fusion. Over 20 Investigational Device Exemption (IDE) studies of spinal arthroplasty were initiated between 2000 and 2020. These studies involved tens of thousands of patients and hundreds of investigational sites, necessarily comparing the investigational arthroplasty devices against a "gold-standard" control fusion procedure. Ultimately, these studies provided a firm evidence basis that cervical and lumbar TDR were, at least, noninferior to their respective fusion comparator groups. Lamentably, the comparison between arthroplasty and fusion continued beyond the FDA regulatory pathway. Even though this regulatory pathway provided strong evidence supporting

Neurosurg Clin N Am 32 (2021) xi–xii
https://doi.org/10.1016/j.nec.2021.07.001
1042-3680/21/© 2021 Published by Elsevier Inc.

the safety and efficacy of these TDR devices in their own right, controversy persisted. Subsequently, the positive results of the early studies have been confirmed with multiple devices with intermediate- and long-term follow-up.[4,5] Although controversy still exists, cervical arthroplasty has been established as a viable alternative to Anterior Cervical Discectomy and Fusion (ACDF) in select patients. The field of spinal arthroplasty remains vibrant and rapidly evolving, and the time has come to move beyond elementary comparisons to fusion. Research needs to focus on refining indications, complication avoidance, and development of next generation devices.[6]

This issue begins with Nunley and Stone providing an overview of the most widely accepted indications and basic technique common to ervical total disc replacement (cTDR). Subsequently, Alves delves into the rationale behind expanding the indications beyond the FDA-approved labeling of cervical arthroplasty. These expanded indications include 3- and 4-level cTDR as well as hybrid TDR and fusion constructs. Bydon and associates describe the cervical devices that have weathered the IDE process and have been granted FDA approval. Guyer and colleagues report on next-generation artificial discs with novel biomaterials and biomechanics as well as the devices that may be next to achieve FDA approval. Rossi and Adamson compare cervical arthroplasty with another motion-preserving procedure, posterior cervical laminoforaminotomy, and discuss the synergy between these approaches. Ray and associates delineate the unique complications associated with cTDR and how best to avoid them. Radcliff and Callahan present and dissect the growing body of long-term level I and II evidence supporting the efficacy of cervical artificial discs. Patwardhan provides an overview of biomechanical considerations associated with the use of arthroplasty in the cervical spine. Coric and Parish discuss the impact of motion preservation on adjacent level reoperation. Franco and associates delineate the history, indications, and evolution of lumbar TDR. Finally, Welch and colleagues examine lumbar arthroplasty from a posterior approach, including artificial facet replacement devices.

Domagoj Coric, MD
Department of Orthopedics
Atrium Healthcare Musculoskeletal Institute
Carolina Neurosurgery and Spine Associates
225 Baldwin Avenue
Charlotte, NC 28204, USA

E-mail address:
dom@cnsa.com

REFERENCES

1. Siemionow K, Hu X, Lieberman I. The Fernstrom ball revisited. Eur Spine J 2012;21:443–8.
2. Büttner-Janz K, Schellnack K, Zippel H. Biomechanics of the SB Charité lumbar intervertebral disc endoprosthesis. Int Orthop 1989;13(3):173–6.
3. Robertson JT, Metcalf NH. Long-term outcome after implantation of the Prestige I disc in an end-stage indication: 4-year results from a pilot study. Neurosurg Focus 2004;17:E10.
4. Garcia R, Zigler J, Radcliff K, et al. Seven-year results of a randomized controlled IDE trial for lumbar artificial discs in single-level degenerative disc. Spine J 2020;20(9):S39–40.
5. Radliff K, Coric D, Albert T. Five-year results of cervical total disc replacement with the Mobi-C cervical artificial disc compared with anterior discectomy and fusion for treatment of 2-level symptomatic degenerative disc disease: an independent critical review of the prospective, randomized, controlled multicenter investigational device exemption clinical trial. J Neurosurg Spine 2016;25(2):1–12.
6. Coric D. Commentary: the effect of T1-slope in spinal parameters after cervical disc arthroplasty. Neurosurgery 2020. nyaa290. doi: 10.1093/neuros/nyaa290.

Cervical Total Disc Replacement: Indications and Technique

Pierce Nunley, MD*, Kelly (Frank) Van Schouwen, MS, Marcus Stone, PhD

KEYWORDS

• Cervical total disc replacement • Cervical indications • Cervical technique

KEY POINTS

• Patient selection for cervical total disc replacement remains a topic of debate among spine surgeons.
• US clinical trials provide the highest level of evidence when analyzing cervical total disc replacement patient selection but are not without some bias.
• Real conditions of use studies should be encouraged to advance the understanding of the best patients to receive cervical disc arthroplasty.

INTRODUCTION

Evidence supporting the use of cervical total disc replacement (cTDR) for treatment of cervical pathology has continued to proliferate since its international adoption in the early 2000s and the first United States (US) Federal Drug Administration (FDA) approval in 2007.[1–3]

While the US was slower to approve and adopt cTDR, the published evidence on its clinical use has outpaced publications from outside the US.[4] In part, the FDA requirements for approval led to this increased body of evidence, as cTDR devices must be studied in an Investigational Device Exemption (IDE) clinical trial to gain FDA approval. The resulting level I evidence including long-term follow-up from these trials is often published, amassing high-quality literature supporting cTDR as a treatment choice.[5–14] Although these studies include level I evidence, they are not without criticism of potential bias.

Historically, the US level I evidence studies have focused on outcomes and complications after treatment of cervical degenerative disc disease with cTDR or anterior cervical discectomy (ACDF). The patient selection for these large-scale US studies was fairly strict, and the surgical technique closely controlled during the IDE trials. The resulting FDA approvals include the specific indications and contraindications for patient selection, and it should be noted that all the trials had very similar and sometimes nearly identical inclusion/exclusion criteria.[1,3,15–24] However, as widespread US clinical use has increased and real-world evidence is collected and published, the importance of tight control of patient selection and surgical technique in clinical practice remains heavily debated.[18,25–29]

Patient selection is not solely a surgeon choice, as there are multiple other controlling variables such as patient anatomy/condition, cost, and insurance. However, it is well documented that patient selection is a key contributing factor to patient outcomes and postoperative complications.[25,30,31]

The cTDR surgical techniques, that were strictly defined and well controlled during clinical trials, are also well documented as contributing factors to patient outcomes and reoperations. Conditions such as heterotopic ossification (HO) and adjacent segment degeneration (ASD) are being studied in more detail, with adjustments to surgical technique and device designs that attempt to minimize these risks.[32–36]

Spine Institute of Louisiana, 1500 Line Avenue, Suite 200, Shreveport, LA 71101, USA
* Corresponding author.
E-mail address: pnunley@louisianaspine.org

Neurosurg Clin N Am 32 (2021) 419–424
https://doi.org/10.1016/j.nec.2021.05.001
1042-3680/21/© 2021 Elsevier Inc. All rights reserved.

Here, we will review the US-approved cTDR patient indications, surgical technique, and the evolution and evidence supporting each. Off-label use and expanded indications for cTDR will be discussed in the next article of this series.

Current United States Patient Indications

The FDA approval of cTDR devices in the US includes specific patient indications and contraindications.[37–47] These patient selection criteria are based on the data collected and analyzed from the IDE clinical trials that supported cTDR approval. If these patient selection criteria are strictly adhered to, it is expected that patient outcomes will mirror the published IDE results.

Currently, there are 9 cTDR devices approved in the US, although not all remain marketed for use. The first cTDRs in the US were both approved in 2007, Prestige ST followed by Prodisc-C (Centinel Spine - West Chester, PA). The Bryan cTDR approval followed shortly after in 2009. Between 2012 and 2020, 6 additional cTDRs received US FDA approval, Secure-C (Globus Medical - Audubon, PA), PCM (NuVasive - SanDiego, CA), Mobi-C (Zimmer Biomet Spine - Warsaw, IN), Prestige LP, M6-C (Orthofix - Lewisville, TX), and Simplify (NuVasive - SanDiego, CA). Both the Mobi-C and Prestige LP (Medtronic - Memphis, TN) received approval for one- and two-level indications, the only current two-level approvals in the US. There are currently no cTDRs indicated for use in greater that 2 contiguous levels, or in conjunction with a previously or concurrently implanted adjacent level ACDF.

While the patient selection criteria for each cTDR vary slightly, there are many similarities that are commonly understood as the accepted criteria (**Box 1**).

As the IDE clinical trials strictly adhered to these criteria, the data available outside of these indications do not meet level I evidence but remain valuable in understand real conditions of use.

Patient selection and outcomes

Improper patient selection has been shown to negatively impact patient outcomes. Some of these negative prognostic factors include disc space collapse greater than 50%, axial neck pain, older patients, preoperative loss of segmental motion, facet arthropathy, osteoporosis, significant kyphosis, segmental instability, trauma, tumor, prior laminectomies, and infection.[27,28,48–51] Patients with these conditions were excluded from IDE clinical trials, but there is now limited real-world evidence published on these patient populations. Although some argue bias within patient selection of IDE clinical trials, the real-world evidence confirms in many cases that these excluded patients may not be good candidates for the currently available cTDR devices.

However, using the strict US selection criteria, it has been demonstrated that less than 50% of patients screened for cTDR are eligible.[26] So, this begs the question, Are there subsets of patients that could benefit from cTDR being excluded?

Design and evolution of cervical total disc replacement—impact to patient selection

While anecdotal, surgeons have indicated for some time that certain cTDR implants may be more suited for certain patients.[51]

Currently, the advances in manufacturing and materials have enabled the design and function of cTDR to evolve with each new device. Initially, cTDR was created in an effort to resolve issues related to motion in the cervical spine. While the gold standard, ACDF, reduced pain, it also removed motion and was suspected to lead to ASD over the long term.

The design of cTDRs has continued to focus on maintenance of motion with the hypothesis that this would also decrease ASD in the long term. The motion allowed by each of the cTDR device designs led to categorize the devices as unconstrained or semiconstrained. However, the literature is conflicting on the classifications of the current cTDRs.[25,52–55]

Generally, the Bryan, Mobi-C, PCM, and Prestige LP have been classified as unconstrained devices. There are reports that indicate the lack of constraint of cTDR could be the cause of hypermobility or sagittal malalignment (ie, kyphosis) in some patients, while other patients experienced spontaneous fusion or HO at the index level.

Prodisc-C, Prestige ST, Simplify, M6, and Secure-C are often considered semi-constrained cTDRs. Similar to unconstrained devices, patients also experienced hypermobility, sagittal malalignment, and HO after surgery with a semiconstrained device.

Diving deeper into the kinematics that surround preservation of motion, Patwardhan and Havey[56] recently reported that understanding a device's degrees of freedom (DOF) and stiffness is more effective in achieving quality of motion, or motion that most closely resembles the natural cervical spine. Using a cTDR with more DOF helps to restore natural motion at a less mobile preoperative segment, while a stiffer construct would restore more natural motion to a patient that presents with a hypermobile preoperative segment. Using the DOF approach is a novel consideration, in lieu of the standard semi-constrained versus constrained classifications.

However, these models do not take into consideration certain anatomic 'normal' variations that exist in the cervical spine. Although of great academic interest, the most important criterion is whether there are measurable and significant clinical outcome differences between the various disc designs. To further confound the issue, do there exist certain anatomic and clinical differences where one implant might work better in one patient versus another?

Currently we are enrolling a level 1 trial with two constrained and one unconstrained device with the intraoperative decision left to the surgeon to choose between the two constrained devices if the patient randomizes to that arm. Data from studies like these will add to the lexicon to help surgeons make more detailed and precise choices for cTDR in the future.

This level of data took 20 to 30 years in the large total joint field, is still being developed in the total ankle and shoulder fields, and likely will take us another decade or two.

As the 3D-printed, patient-specific implants continue to advance, perhaps these are a future consideration for clinical trials to expand cTDR indications and possibilities for patient-specific implants that could further positively impact patient outcomes.

Surgical Technique

The general surgical technique for cTDR is well established, while there are some additional techniques and tips that are based on the specific cTDR being implanted. The general surgical steps, with additional tips, are outlined in the following section.

The Smith-Robinson approach is first used to access the anterior cervical spine.

Soft-tissue retraction can be accomplished manually with handheld retractors or using one of various 'self-retaining' retractor systems tucked under the longus colli muscles.

Distraction pins are placed in the mid-vertebral bodies cranial and caudal to the disc space and gentle distraction applied. It is important not to overdistract or implant a cTDR device that is too large (specifically height) for the diseased segment, as this has been shown to result in negative patient outcomes. However, Patwardan and Havey recently reported that patients with less than 3 mm of disc height could potentially be treated with a compressible disc that would avoid overdistracting.[56]

After gentle distraction, anterior discectomy and decompression are completed, with decompression of the uncovertebral joints bilaterally.

Release of the posterior longitudinal ligament (PLL) is the surgeon's discretion and may also depend on the type of cTDR being implanted. There are varied opinions on the value of preserving or resecting the PLL. Preservation of the PLL is hypothesized to maintain appropriate range of motion (ROM) versus causing hypermobility when resected.[57,58] However, prior studies indicate that hypermobility appears to be overcome with implantation of a "stiffer" cTDR.[59] Surgeons that support resection of the PLL report it is the best way to ensure that an adequate decompression is achieved.

After the decision to resect or retain the PLL, osteophytes are removed, and the end plates are prepped for the implant. The preparation of end plates can be minimal, exposing underlying bone only, or more involved if the device contains a keel that must be cut into the endplate.

One of the most important areas to focus decompression is the posterior uncovertebral joints as they form the proximal aspect of the neuroforamen. Any neuroforaminal stenosis in the area must be decompressed to decompress the exiting nerve root and prevent nerve root irritation postoperatively when the patient moves their neck.

Whether to use a power burr is vigorously debated among experts. There are also regional and training differences. The debate is whether to get a better fit and possibly slightly larger footprint versus the risk of HO. However, to date, there has been nothing definitively published to relate burring to the presence of HO. Furthermore, even in our own research and publications, we have essentially shown that HO is not a 'clinical' syndrome, and there are no significant outcome differences between those patients that developed HO versus those that did not, outside of the lost ROM at the segment.[60] Finally, there is some literature to suggest that more coverage of the implant decreases HO. Therefore, it would be reasonable to slightly burr the uncus to get a larger foot print device implanted if it gives better coverage and all the other parameters are within limits.

Trialing is then completed to determine the proper implant sizing. This should be checked on anterior-posterior (AP) and lateral imaging. Many patients will have asymmetry in the uncus, and although the disc may 'look' midline, it could be shifted laterally. In these situations, either choose a smaller implant that can be centered or use a burr that could carefully remove the intruding uncus so that the trial may be centered with appropriate endplate apposition.

For devices that require keel cuts, this is accomplished next per the manufacturers' guidelines.

The cTDR is then impacted in the disc space using fluoroscopic imaging to assess appropriate placement. Finally, distraction is released and many recommend a gentle 'squeezing' of the pins to 'set' the device. Placement of the cTDR is confirmed with AP and lateral fluoroscopy, and minor adjustments are made as needed.

Each cTDR device has some surgical techniques that are specific to its design and are not mentioned in detail previously. Leven and colleagues, 2017, detail the surgical technique for most cTDRs currently available in the US.[51]

Given these subtle differences between surgical techniques, it is important to consider the significance of surgeon training to each cTDR device. A key part of the US IDE clinical trials was extensive training to the cTDR surgical technique. In addition, most trials included a training case for each surgeon. After obtaining FDA approval, the national release of a cTDR device included surgeon training, but the increased volume of use would be difficult to control the surgical technique to the same level as was achieved during the clinical trial. Therefore, it is expected that real-world use of cTDR could result in higher complication rates related to surgical technique, particularly during early adoption.

SUMMARY

We acknowledge that patient selection during clinical trials may contain some bias, although currently the published real conditions of use studies available support many of these selection criteria to ensure the best possible outcomes for patients treated with cTDR. We encourage further real conditions of use studies to continue to understand the best patient selection for cTDR.

Surgical technique remains critical to patient success after cTDR surgery. Evidence suggests that avoiding overdistraction remains a key factor, while the debate to maintain or resect the PLL and the judicious use of a power burr may not be as critical as previously thought.

CLINICS CARE POINTS

- A conservative approach to surgical indications could eliminate potential benefits to some patients.
- The various cervical total disc replacement designs should be evaluated for potential benefits when selected to accommodate specific patient indications.
- Real conditions of use studies are important to understand the risks/benefits when used outside highly controlled clinical trials and to grow overall adoption of cervical total disc replacement.

DISCLOSURE

All disclosures are related to cervical total disc replacements. P. Nunley and M. Stone have received consulting fees from Simplify Medical. K.V. Schouwen has no relevant disclosures.

REFERENCES

1. US Food and Drug Administration. Summary of Safety and Effectiveness data (SSED): prodisc-C

total disc replacement. Washington, DC: US Food and Drug Administration; 2007.

2. Bryan VE. Cervical motion segment replacement. Eur Spine J 2002;11(SUPPL. 2).

3. US Food and Drug Administration. Summary of Safety and Effectiveness data (SSED). Washington, DC: Bryan Cervical Disc.; 2007.

4. Nunley PD, Coric D, Frank KA, et al. Cervical Disc Arthroplasty: Current Evidence and Real-World Application. Clin Neurosurg 2018;83(6):1087–106.

5. Bae H, Nunley P, Davis R, et al. One-Level vs. Two-Level Treatment for Cervical Total Disc Replacement and Anterior Cervical Discectomy and Fusion at 7-year Follow-up (Podium). In: International meeting on advanced spine techniques (IMAST). Washington DC, 13-16 July 2016.

6. Radcliff K, Davis RJ, Hisey MS, et al. Long-term Evaluation of Cervical Disc Arthroplasty with the Mobi-C©Cervical Disc: A Randomized, Prospective, Multicenter Clinical Trial with Seven-Year Follow-up. Int J Spine Surg [Internet] 2017;11(4):31.

7. Davis RJ, Nunley PD, Kim KD, et al. Two-level total disc replacement with Mobi-C cervical artificial disc versus anterior discectomy and fusion: A prospective, randomized, controlled multicenter clinical trial with 4-year follow-up results. J Neurosurg Spine 2015;22(1):15–25.

8. Hisey M, Bae H, Davis R, et al. One-level Treatment with Total Disc Replacement and ACDF: Results from an FDA IDE Clinical Trial through 60 Months (Podium). In: International Society for the Advancement of spine surgery (ISASS). Washington DC, 13-16 July 2016.

9. Pandey PK, Pawar I, Gupta J, et al. Comparison of Outcomes of Single-Level Anterior Cervical Discectomy With Fusion and Single- Level Artificial Cervical Disc Replacement for Single-Level Cervical Degenerative Disc Disease. Spine (Phila Pa 1976) 2017;42(1).

10. Gornet MF, Lanman TH, Burkus JK, et al. Cervical disc arthroplasty with the Prestige LP disc versus anterior cervical discectomy and fusion, at 2 levels: results of a prospective, multicenter randomized controlled clinical trial at 24 months. J Neurosurg Spine [Internet 2017;26(6):653–67.

11. Coric D, Parish J, Boltes MO. M6-C artificial disc placement. Neurosurg Focus. Am Assoc Neurol Surgeons 2017;42:1.

12. Phillips FM, Geisler FH, Gilder KM, et al. Long-term outcomes of the US FDA IDE prospective, randomized controlled clinical trial comparing PCM cervical disc arthroplasty with anterior cervical discectomy and fusion. Spine (Phila Pa 1976) 2015;40(10):674–83.

13. Upadhyaya CD, Wu JC, Trost G, et al. Analysis of the three united states food and drug administration investigational device exemption cervical arthroplasty trials: Clinical article. J Neurosurg Spine 2012 Mar;16(3):216–28.

14. Janssen ME, Zigler JE, Spivak JM, et al. ProDisc-C Total Disc Replacement Versus Anterior Cervical Discectomy and Fusion for Single-Level Symptomatic Cervical Disc Disease: Seven-Year Follow-up of the Prospective Randomized U.S. Food and Drug Administration Investigational Device Exemption Study. J Bone Jt Surg Am [Internet] 2015;97(21):1738–47.

15. US Food and Drug Administration. Summary of Safety and Effectiveness data (SSED): M6 cervical disc replacement. Washington, DC: US Food and Drug Administration; 2019.

16. US Food and Drug Administration. Summary of Safety and Effectiveness data (SSED): Simplify cervical disc. Washington, DC: US Food and Drug Administration; 2020.

17. US Food and Drug Administration. Summary of Safety and Effectivness (SSED): Prestige LP cervical disc - 1-level. Washington, DC: US Food and Drug Administration; 2016.

18. Nunley P, Frank K, Stone M. Patient selection in cervical disc arthroplasty. Int J Spine Surg 2020;14(s2):S29–35.

19. US Food and Drug Administration. Summary of Safety and Effectiveness (SSED): Prestige LP cervical disc - 2-level. Washington, DC: US Food and Drug Administration; 2014.

20. US Food and Drug Administration. Summary of Safety and Effectiveness data (SSED): Mobi-C cervical disc Prosthesis - 1-level. Washington, DC: US Food and Drug Administration; 2013.

21. US Food and Drug Administration. Summary of Safety and Effectiveness (SSED): Mobi-C cervical disc Prosthesis 2-level. Washington, DC: US Food and Drug Administration; 2013.

22. US Food and Drug Administration. Summary of Safety and Effectiveness data (SSED). Washington, DC: US Food and Drug Administration; 2012.

23. US Food and Drug Administration. Summary of Safety and Effectiveness data (SSED). Washington, DC: US Food and Drug Administration; 2012.

24. US Food and Drug Administration. Summary of Safety and Effectiveness data (SSED): Prestige cervical disc. Washington, DC: US Food and Drug Administration; 2016.

25. Park CK, Ryu KS. Are controversial issues in cervical total disc replacement resolved or unresolved?: A review of literature and recent updates. Asian Spine J Korean Soc Spine Surg 2018;12:178–92.

26. Auerbach JD, Jones KJ, Fras CI, et al. The prevalence of indications and contraindications to cervical total disc replacement. Spine J 2008;8(5):711–6.

27. Gelalis ID, Papadopoulos DV, Giannoulis DK, et al. Spinal motion preservation surgery: indications and applications. Vol. 28, European Journal of Orthopaedic surgery and Traumatology. France: Springer-Verlag; 2018. p. 335–42.

28. Salari B, McAfee PC. Cervical Total Disk Replacement: Complications and Avoidance. Orthop Clin North Am 2012;43:97–107.

29. Turel MK, Kerolus MG, Adogwa O, et al. Cervical arthroplasty: What does the labeling say? Neurosurg Focus 2017;42(2).

30. Passias PG, Hasan S, Radcliff K, et al. Arm pain versus neck pain: A novel ratio as a predictor of post-operative clinical outcomes in cervical radiculopathy patients. Int J Spine Surg 2018;12(5):638–43.

31. Sasso WR, Smucker JD, Sasso MP, et al. Long-term Clinical Outcomes of Cervical Disc Arthroplasty: A Prospective, Randomized, Controlled Trial. Spine (Phila Pa 1976) 2017;42(4):209–16.

32. Pimenta L, Oliveira L, Coutinho E, et al. Bone formation in cervical total disk replacement (CTDR) up to the 6-year follow-up. Neurosurg Quart 2013;23:1–6.

33. Cho Y-H, Kim K-S, Kwon Y-M. Heterotopic ossification after cervical arthroplasty with ProDisc-C: time Course Radiographic follow-up over 3 years Corresponding [Internet], vol. 10. Korean J Spine; 2013. Available at: www.e-kjs.org.

34. Chang P-Y, Wu J-C, Mayo BC, et al. Heterotopic Ossification in Cervical Disc Arthroplasty. Contemp Spine Surg 2017;18(5):1–5.

35. Nunley PD, Kerr EJ, Cavanaugh DA, et al. Adjacent segment pathology after treatment with cervical disc arthroplasty or anterior cervical discectomy and fusion, part 2: Clinical results at 7-year follow-up. Int J Spine Surg 2020;14(3):278–85.

36. Nunley PD, Kerr EJ, Cavanaugh DA, et al. Adjacent segment pathology after treatment with cervical disc arthroplasty or anterior cervical discectomy and fusion, part 1: Radiographic results at 7-year follow-up. Int J Spine Surg 2020;14(3):269–77.

37. US Food and Drug Administration. Product labeling for Prestige cervical disc. Washington, DC: US Food and Drug Administration; 2007.

38. US Food and Drug Administration. Product labeling for M6-CTM Artificial cervical disc. Washington, DC: US Food and Drug Administration; 2019.

39. US Food and Drug Administration. Product labeling for PCM cervical disc. Washington, DC: US Food and Drug Administration; 2012.

40. US Food and Drug Administration. Product labeling for Simplify ® cervical Artificial disc. Washington, DC: US Food and Drug Administration; 2020.

41. US Food and Drug Administration. Product labeling for Prodisc-C cervical disc. Washington, DC: US Food and Drug Administration; 2007.

42. US Food and Drug Administration. Product labeling for Bryan cervical disc. Washington, DC: US Food and Drug Administration; 2009.

43. US Food and Drug Administration. Product labeling for Secure-C cervical disc. Washington, DC: US Food and Drug Administration; 2012.

44. US Food and Drug Administration. Product labeling for Mobi-C cervical disc. Washington, DC: US Food and Drug Administration; 2013.

45. US Food and Drug Administration. Product labeling for Mobi-C (2-level) cervical disc. Washington, DC: US Food and Drug Administration; 2013.

46. US Food and Drug Administration. Product labeling for Prestige-LP (2-level) cervical disc 2016. Washington, DC.

47. US Food and Drug Administration. Product labeling for Prestige-LP (1-level) cervical disc. Washington, DC: US Food and Drug Administration; 2014.

48. Ding D, Shaffrey ME. Cervical Disk Arthroplasty: Patient Selection. Clin Neurosurg 2012;59:91–7.

49. Tu TH, Wu JC, Huang WC, et al. Heterotopic ossification after cervical total disc replacement: Determination by CT and effects on clinical outcomes. Clinical article. J Neurosurg Spine 2011;14(4):457–65.

50. McAfee PC. The indications for lumbar and cervical disc replacement. Spine J 2004;4(6 SUPPL):S177–81.

51. Leven D, Meaike J, Radcliff K, et al. Cervical disc replacement surgery: indications, technique, and technical pearls. Curr Rev Musculoskelet Med 2017;10(2):160–9.

52. Choi H, Baisden JL, Yoganandan N. A comparative in vivo study of semi-constrained and unconstrained cervical artificial disc prostheses. Mil Med 2019;184(Suppl 1):637–43.

53. Sekhon LHS, Ball JR. Artificial cervical disc replacement: principles, types and techniques. Neurol India 2005;53(4):445–50.

54. Vaccaro A, Beutler W, Peppelman W, et al. Long-term clinical experience with selectively constrained SECURE-C cervical artificial disc for 1-level cervical disc disease: Results from seven-year follow-up of a prospective, randomized, controlled investigational device exemption clinical trial. Int J Spine Surg 2018;12(3):377–87.

55. Sundseth J, Jacobsen EA, Kolstad F, et al. Heterotopic ossification and clinical outcome in nonconstrained cervical arthroplasty 2 years after surgery: the Norwegian Cervical Arthroplasty Trial (NORCAT). Eur Spine J [Internet] 2016;25(7):2271–8.

56. Patwardhan AG, Havey RM. Biomechanics of Cervical Disc Arthroplasty—A Review of Concepts and Current Technology. Int J Spine Surg 2020;14(s2):S14–28.

57. Lazaro BCR, Yucesoy K, Yuksel KZ, et al. Effect of arthroplasty design on cervical spine kinematics: Analysis of the Bryan disc, ProDisc-C, and Synergy disc. Neurosurg Focus 2010;28(6):1–8.

58. Kim SW, Paik S-H, Castro PAF, et al. Analysis of factors that may influence range of motion after cervical disc arthroplasty. Spine J 2010;10(8).

59. Voronov LI, Havey RM, Tsitsopoulos PP, et al. Does resection of the posterior longitudinal ligament affect the stability of cervical disc arthroplasty? Int J Spine Surg 2018;12(2):285–94.

60. Nunley PD, Cavanaugh DA, Kerr EJ, et al. Heterotopic ossification after cervical total disc replacement at 7 years-prevalence, progression, clinical implications, and risk factors. Int J Spine Surg 2018;12(3):352–61.

Cervical Total Disc Replacement
Food and Drug Administration–Approved Devices

Mohamad Bydon, MD[a,b,c],*, Giorgos D. Michalopoulos, MD[a,b,c],
Mohammed Ali Alvi, MBBS, MS[a,b,c], Anshit Goyal, MBBS, MS[a,b,c],
Kingsley Abode-Iyamah, MD[d]

KEYWORDS

- FDA-approved artificial discs • Single-level CTDR • Two-level CTDR

KEY POINTS

- Nine artificial discs have been approved by the US Food and Drug Administration (FDA) for single-level cervical total disc replacement (CTDR):PRESTIGE ST, PRODISC-C, BRYAN, SECURE-C, PCM, Mobi-C, PRESTIGE LP, M6-C, and Simplify.
- Mobi-C and PRESTIGE LP have been approved for 2-level CTDR.
- FDA Investigational Device Exemption trials have shown noninferiority of CTDR compared with anterior cervical decompression and fusion.

INTRODUCTION

The gold-standard surgical treatment of patients with cervical radiculopathy or myelopathy caused by disc herniation or spondylosis has traditionally been anterior cervical decompression and fusion (ACDF); however, restricted mobility and concerns related to adjacent segment disease (ASD) led to the development of a motion-preserving alternative. Cervical total disc replacement (CTDR) offers a suitable alternative for carefully selected patients, which allows resolution of compressive disorder while preserving segmental motion.

At present, the Food and Drug Administration (FDA) in the United States has approved the commercial distribution of 9 CTDR devices (**Table 1**), arranged here in chronologic order of FDA approval:

- PRESTIGE ST (Medtronic Sofamor Danek, Memphis, TN)[a]
- PRODISC-C (Centinel Spine, West Chester, PA)
- BRYAN (Medtronic Sofamor Danek, Memphis, TN)[a]
- SECURE-C (Globus Medical, Audubon, PA)
- PCM (NuVasive Inc, San Diego, CA)
- Mobi-C (LDR, Sainte-Savine, France)
- PRESTIGE LP (Medtronic Sofamor Danek, Memphis, TN)
- M6-C (Spinal Kinetics, Sunnyvale, CA)
- Simplify (Simplify Medical, Sunnyvale, CA)

This article describes the path to FDA approval for CTDR, discusses the salient features of approved CTDR devices, and presents a comparison of clinically relevant parameters among these approved devices.

[a] Mayo Clinic Neuro-Informatics Laboratory, Mayo Clinic, Rochester, MN 55902, USA; [b] Department of Neurologic Surgery, Mayo Clinic, Rochester, MN 55902, USA; [c] Department of Neurosurgery, Mayo Clinic, 200 First Street Southwest, Rochester, MN, USA; [d] Department of Neurosurgery, Mayo Clinic, 4500 San Pablo Road, Jacksonville, FL 32224, USA
* Corresponding author. Department of Neurosurgery, Mayo Clinic, 200 First Street Southwest, Rochester, MN.
E-mail address: bydon.mohamad@mayo.edu

[a]No longer manufactured for distribution.

Neurosurg Clin N Am 32 (2021) 425–435
https://doi.org/10.1016/j.nec.2021.05.003
1042-3680/21/© 2021 Elsevier Inc. All rights reserved.

Table 1
US Food and Drug Administration–approved artificial discs for 1-level cervical total disc replacement until October 2020

Device	Material	Characteristics
PRESTIGE ST	Stainless steel	Ball in trough, Large prevertebral fixation system
PRODISC-C[a]	CoCrMo endplates, UHMWPE core	Ball and socket, fixed center of rotation
BRYAN	Ti endplates, PU nucleus and shell	Shock-absorbing potential, unconstrained
SECURE-C	CoCrMo endplates, UHMWPE core	Ball in trough, semiconstrained, translation enabled
PCM	CoCrMo endplates, UHMWPE core	Ball and socket, unconstrained
Mobi-C	CoCrMo endplates, UHMWPE core	Ball in trough, unconstrained, translation in 2 planes. Also, 2-level approved
PRESTIGE LP	Ti ceramic	Ball in trough, semiconstrained, translation enabled. Also, 2-level approved
M6-C	Ti endplates, PU nucleus, UHMWPE annulus	Shock-absorbing properties, 6° of freedom
Simplify	PEEK endplates, ceramic core	Translation in 2 planes

Abbreviations: CoCrMo, cobalt, chromium, molybdenum; PEEK, polyether ether ketone; PU, polyurethane; Ti, titanium; UHMWPE, ultrahigh-molecular-weight polyethylene.
[a] The original PRODISC-C device.

FOOD AND DRUG ADMINISTRATION APPROVAL PROCESS

CTDR devices are considered class III devices by the FDA; that is, "those that support or sustain human life, are of substantial importance in preventing impairment of human health, or which present a potential, unreasonable risk of illness or injury."[1] Thus, these devices are subject to stringent evaluation before they are made available, a process designed to obtain premarket approval (PMA).

Most devices are initially implanted in cadaveric models and tested on mechanical parameters, such as range of motion and alignment. This testing is usually followed by some single-arm feasibility clinical studies with a brief follow-up period of no more than 2 years, which provides a vague measure of efficacy for a small number of eligible patients, while concomitantly providing a first impression of the risks and adverse events. Most of the aforementioned devices went through the latter phase in Europe.

A critical step for PMA is a multicenter FDA Investigational Device Exemption (IDE) randomized clinical trial (RCT). In such a trial, the FDA allows the use of the device in limited centers and sets the regulations under which CTDR with the investigated device will be compared with ACDF,

the existing gold standard. The primary aim of these trials is usually to establish safety and efficacy with a noninferiority statistical design. The patients are randomized to either procedure type, are not blinded because of the nature of the intervention, and are generally followed for 10 years. The primary outcome is overall success (defined later), whereas common secondary outcomes include Neck Disability Index (NDI), visual analog scale pain score, and rates of ASD and reoperation. Noninferiority results compared with ACDF at the end of 2-year follow-up are usually sufficient to grant PMA.

FDA-approved devices are then allowed to be manufactured and marketed; however, the IDE study sponsor is required to follow the study cohort for 7 to 10 years in total and report to the FDA long-term outcomes annually, even following PMA. So far, only the PRESTIGE and BRYAN devices have gone through the entire 10-year postapproval process.

The overall success of both ACDF and CTDR, which is the primary end point of the FDA IDE trials so far, is defined as the fulfillment of a composite measure, typically consisting of the following criteria:

1. Improvement of more than 15 points in the NDI scale compared with preoperative status.

2. Maintenance or improvement of the neurologic status.[2]
3. No grade III or IV adverse events related to the procedure or the implant.
4. No subsequent operation or intervention classified as failure.[3]

In some clinical trials, a fifth criterion, requiring no intraoperative treatment change, is also added.[4]

PER DEVICE ANALYSIS
PRESTIGE ST

PRESTIGE ST was the first CTDR device to be approved by the FDA for market distribution in the United States, in July 2007.[5] It was approved for 1-level cervical arthroplasty from C3 to C7 for cases of symptomatic myelopathy or radiculopathy.

The PRESTIGE ST is a 2-piece, ball-in-trough, semiconstrained, noncompressible stainless steel device. Its distinguishing characteristic is its sizable fixation components. The device is secured by 4 screws (2 for each vertebral body) and a locking mechanism to keep the screws in place.

It was tested in an FDA IDE RCT, where the control arm was treated with ACDF. The trial started in 2002 and early results were published in 2007 by Mummaneni and colleagues.[6] The data from this cohort showed superiority of CTDR compared with ACDF in overall success rates (75% vs 63.7%; $P = .008$) after 84 months of follow-up.[6] Notably, the rate of reoperation for adjacent-level disease was 2.5 times greater (4.6% vs 11.9%; $P = .008$) in the ACDF arm. Slightly more than 1 in 10 cases of CTDR were complicated by dysphonia or dysphagia being present at the 7-year follow-up, a rate almost equal to that observed in the ACDF group. The PRESTIGE ST is no longer manufactured because it was replaced by the PRESTIGE LP; nevertheless, it represented a significant milestone as the first cervical arthroplasty device to receive FDA approval.

PRODISC-C

The PRODISC-C is a 3-piece, noncompressible ball-and-socket device: the 2 endplates are made of a cobalt–chromium-molybdenum (CoCrMo) alloy and are separated by an ultrahigh-molecular-weight polyethylene (UHMWPE) layer. The latter is fixated on the upper surface of the lower endplate and comprises the ball that enters the socket; that is, the cavity in the lower surface of the upper endplate. In terms of mobility, the device is considered semiconstrained, with a fixed center of rotation.[7]

The design used to accommodate fixation of the device on the vertebral bodies includes 2 flat, titanium-sprayed surfaces with a long keel on each of them. The continuous keel is characteristic and may be used to distinguish PRODISC-C from the other 8 artificial discs described in this article on an anteroposterior or posteroanterior cervical spine radiograph. The keel of the SECURE-C is not continuous, which is noticeable in a lateral radiograph.

There are 2 more models of PRODISC-C, Vivo and SK, neither of which is currently available in the US market. They are both mainly made of titanium alloy, containing a CoCrMo alloy calotte insert and a core similar to the original PRODISC-C disc.

The first clinical single-arm trial using PRODISC-C was published in 2005.[8] By this time, an FDA IDE had already been initiated. The results of the corresponding RCT showed noninferiority of the CTDR group compared with the ACDF group during the entire 7-year follow-up, and even superiority with regard to reoperation rate: in the 7-year follow-up publication, this rate is one-fifth of the reoperation rate following ACDF.[9–11] This feature stood out in analogous trials for approval of the other 2 early devices, and, diachronically, it is portrayed to be a significant advantage of CTDR.

The 2 arms of this RCT in the 7-year follow-up were also compared based on cost-effectiveness: the PRODISC-C group was significantly superior to ACDF, resulting in cost-savings of $12,000 per patient while having a higher quality-adjusted life year score.[12] To our knowledge, there are no studies comparing cost-effectiveness between different artificial disc models; hence, all comparisons in this article have been made with ACDF. The PRODISC-C was approved by the FDA for 1-level C3-C7 CTDR in skeletally mature patients in December 2007 (**Fig. 1**).[13] In 2019, another FDA trial started, this time evaluating the performance of both Vivo and SK in CTDR of 2 contiguous levels versus the performance of Mobi-C, an FDA-approved device for 2-level operations that is discussed later.

BRYAN

This device received FDA approval in May 2009 for single-level C3-C7 CTDR in patients with cervical myelopathy and/or radiculopathy.[14,15] It is an unconstrained 4-component artificial disc: 1 polyurethane nucleus surrounded perimetrically by a polyurethane outer shell and covered above and below by titanium endplates. The surfaces that

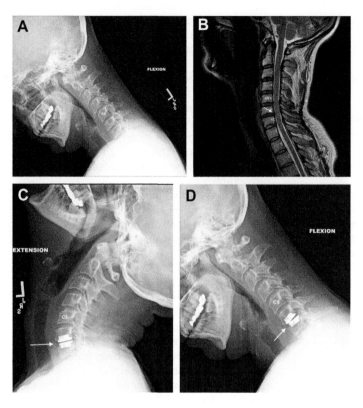

Fig. 1. A 43-year-old female patient presented with a 2-month history of cervicalgia and left C7 radiculopathy. (*A*) Preoperative cervical spine radiograph. C6-C7 disc herniation was seen on MRI of the cervical spine (*B*). Single-level CTDR of C6-C7 disc with Prodisc-C was performed in extension (*C*), and in flexion (*D*). Artificial disc shows significant increase in disc height (*white arrow*) in flexion compared with (*A*).

contact the bone are covered by a titanium porous coating to provide friction and stable integration. There are small vertical protrusions in the anterior part of the disc to prevent the dorsal migration of the implant and to facilitate its removal; these protrusions are characteristic of this particular device in lateral cervical spine radiographs. The polyurethane core potentially offers absorption of vertical forces. The BRYAN device differs from most of the other devices in that deep milling of the vertebral bone is required for its stabilization, which increases the surgical complexity and exposes a significant amount of cancellous bone.[7]

The first systematic clinical application of BRYAN was in a study from Belgium that showed clear improvement in patient status compared with the preoperative baseline, and a reassuring safety profile.[16] Two-level procedures were also included in this trial. An IDE was cleared by the FDA, and an RCT using an ACDF comparison group took place in multiple hospitals from 2002 to 2004.[17] The results were satisfactory enough for the device to be granted FDA approval: CTDR with BRYAN performed better than ACDF in terms of overall success and postoperative NDI scores throughout the 10-year follow-up and maintained an average angle of motion of 8.7°, which was 2.2° more than the analogous preoperative value.[18]

There have been some trials on 2-level operations, with varying results; however, none of the studies had a sufficient sample size or adequate follow-up to receive FDA approval for this indication.[19–21]

SECURE-C

SECURE-C is a 3-piece, ball-in-trough cervical disc: it consists of 2 CoCrMo alloy endplates and an UHMWPE core with protuberances that insert into cavities within the endplates. As far as functionality is concerned, the upper protuberance is spherical, allowing rotation in all 3 planes, whereas the lower is cylindrical, restricting rotatory motion in the coronal and transverse planes. Axial rotation is unconstrained; that is, it is limited by ligaments and the posterior elements. Fixation is achieved by a noncontinuous keel, which is characteristically depicted in a lateral radiograph.

The device was approved by the FDA in September 2012 for use in skeletally mature patients in 1-level CTDR between C3 and C7.[22] The trial that justified this decision had its first results published in 2013,[4] which showed superiority of CTDR compared with ACDF in overall success, as well as in some secondary end points. These results were confirmed in the 7-year follow-up.[23] The device was never subjected to an FDA-directed performance evaluation for 2-level operations.

PCM

PCM is an unconstrained ball-and-socket device, consisting of 2 CoCrMo alloy endplates and an UHMWPE core attached to the lower endplate. The coating is porous (the acronym PCM stands for porous coating motion) and made of titanium and calcium phosphate. In terms of motion, PCM allows for translation because of the size of the ball-and-socket formation.

The initial clinical investigations took place in Brazil, where approximately half of the patients received a 2-level or 3-level CTDR, with promising results.[24] The same Brazilian center reported 71 additional 2-level cases,[25] with excellent or good outcomes in 85% of cases based on the original criteria described by Odom and colleagues.[26] Nonetheless, the device never underwent an FDA-guided randomized controlled trial for 2-level procedures, and, hence, was never approved. As far as single-level CTDR is concerned, PCM was approved by the FDA in October 2012, following a typical FDA IDE RCT comparing the operation with ACDF.[27,28] Once again, CTDR proved noninferior in every investigated parameter (including overall success), and even superiority in some patient-reported satisfaction scales.[29] Interestingly, this was the first IDE trial to include patients with a history of prior ACDF undergoing CTDR at an adjacent level, as well as disc replacement at the C7-T1 level. Neither of these 2 expanded indications of PCM received FDA approval.

Mobi-C

Mobi-C is a 3-piece, ball-in-trough artificial disc. Its metallic endplates are made of CoCrMo alloy and the core is made of UHMWPE. The caudal surface of the cranial endplate has a spherical evagination, in which the core articulates. Every movement of the cranial endplate applies forces with different directions to the core, resulting in its movement relative to the caudal endplate. The movement is constrained by metal bars in the lateral regions of the device. The coating is an alloy of titanium and hydroxyapatite and fixation is further empowered by lateral spikes. Functionally, the device is designed to allow both anteroposterior and lateral translation, which is independent from rotatory movement. This design supposedly results in 5 independent degrees of motion.[30]

The first robust evidence to support its use came from France, where Mobi-C had been used for 1-level and 2-level procedures since 2004.[31] The device was subjected to the typical FDA approval process for both single-level and double-level CTDR, comparing it with the equivalent ACDF operations. The results of the 2-year follow-up of these 2 IDE RCTs were published in 2013 and 2014.[30,32] For 1-level CTDR versus ACDF, the investigational arm achieved noninferiority in rates of overall success as well as secondary end points. For 2-level surgeries, the results were even more encouraging, because the investigated group performed superiorly to the standard-of-care procedure in terms of overall success (60.8% vs 34.2%; $P<.0001$), as well as rates of ASD (50.7% vs 90.5%; $P<.0001$).[3,33] The device was approved in August 2013 for 1-level and 2-contiguous-level CTDR in skeletally mature patients for C3-C7 levels.[34,35] It was the first time an artificial disc received clearance for 2-level implantation. Cost-effectiveness for 2-level CTDR versus ACDF was evaluated at 5-year follow-up. Although the initial cost of the investigational arthroplasty group was almost $2000 higher, when loss of productivity and return-to-work rates were included in the economic analysis, the arthroplasty group was shown to be more cost-effective.[36]

PRESTIGE LP

This newer PRESTIGE model consists of 2 endplates interfacing in a ball-in-trough fashion, a feature unique among the newer FDA-approved artificial discs, which tend to use a polyethylene core to separate the 2 metallic surfaces.

The endplates of PRESTIGE LP are not metallic per se: they are made of a titanium ceramic composite that contains traces of aluminum and vanadium; thus, it is a safe choice for patients that are hypersensitive to the more commonly used metals chrome and nickel. The fixation mechanism uses the commonly used titanium spray coating, along with 2 serrated rails on each endplate. The presence of these rails, when combined with the lack of radiolucent material between the endplates, can be used for a fairly certain recognition of this particular device in a cervical spine radiograph. From a kinematic perspective, this artificial disc belongs in the broad category of semiconstrained discs: it is unconstrained in the axial plain but allows finite coronal rotation (ie, flexion-extension) and translation, the latter of which is enabled by the imperfect articulation between the male and the female parts of the device that allows their relative movements.

The device was evaluated in 2 separate IDE clinical trials: 1 for 1-level CTDR, and another for 2-level CTDR. In 1-level operations, PRESTIGE LP CTDR performance was statistically noninferior or superior to ACDF, depending on which overall success criteria were used.[28] Methodologically, this clinical trial contains the peculiarity of using as a control arm the ACDF cohort from the RCT for the approval of PRESTIGE ST, in lieu of recruiting new patients. The device was approved by the FDA for 1-level CTDR in skeletally mature patients for the levels C3 to C7 in July 2014.[37] The second IDE trial showed statistically significant superiority of the 2-level CTDR compared with 2-level ACDF in overall success, NDI improvement, and neurologic outcome.[38,39] Economic analysis of the results of both 1-level and 2-level CTDR showed similar cost-effectiveness to ACDF.[40,41]

Overall, there are several contradicting articles on whether CTDR is more cost-effective than ACDF; the general pattern among them is that they are at least equal, and the superiority of CTDR is more evident as the follow-up period increases, because of fewer late-onset complications and reoperations.[36,40,42,43] Also, most investigators agree that CTDR correlates with faster return to work and better quality of life.[12,40,42] The FDA issued the approval for CTDR using PRESTIGE LP in skeletally mature patients at 2 adjacent levels between C3 and C7 in July 2016 (**Fig. 2**).[44]

M6-C

The idea behind the design of this artificial device is to simulate the properties of a natural intervertebral disc with components mimicking both the annulus fibrosus and the nucleus pulposus. The 2 endplates are made of titanium and their fixation to the vertebrae is accommodated by serrated keels and porous titanium spray on the contact surfaces. The unique core is composed of a compressible polyurethane nucleus surrounded by a weave of ultrahigh-molecular-weight polyethylene fibers. The annulus fibers are bound to the endplates. The device is claimed to give 6° of freedom of motion and compressible properties.

M6-C was initially CE (Conformité Européenne) marked and used in Europe in 2005 and initiated an IDE pilot 1-armed feasibility study 3 years later. This trial was preceded by a few similar studies abroad, namely in Mexico and Belgium, which found M6-C to be safe and effective.[45,46] This finding was confirmed by the IDE trial, which included only 30 patients, most of whom underwent a 2-level CTDR. After 2 years of follow-up, the overall success rate of the CTDR was 89%.[31] The device subsequently underwent a full IDE trial with M6-C compared with a concurrent, nonrandomized ACDF cohort, which ultimately led to FDA approval in February 2019.[47] In this propensity-matched multi-institutional trial, the success rate of the M6-C group (86.8%) was non-inferior to the respective rate for ACDF (79.3%), while the M6-C group demonstrated greater improvement in quality-of-life and pain scores.[48]

Simplify

This device is the latest addition to the list of the FDA-approved artificial discs. Simplify was granted permission for market distribution in September 2020; it is indicated for 1-level CTDR at levels C3 to C7 in skeletally mature patients with radiculopathy or myelopathy.[49]

It is constituted by 2 endplates made of polyether ether ketone (PEEK) and a biconvex zirconia toughened alumina ceramic core between them. Fixation to the vertebral body is secured by serrated keels and titanium spray. Overall, this device contains the least metal among those previously discussed, potentially signifying the highest MRI compatibility. From a kinematic perspective, the core is limited by a retention ring that allows translation in any direction, and the device is supposed to enable flexion-extension range of motion up to 12°.

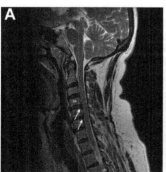
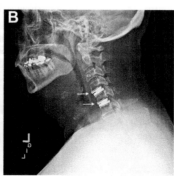

Fig. 2. A 51-year-old woman presented with a 4-month history of C5 and C6 radiculopathy without signs of myelopathy, following motor vehicle collision. MRI of the cervical spine showed disc herniation at C4-C5 and C5-C6 levels (A, white arrows). She underwent 2-level CTDR at the levels of disorder with PRESTIGE LP (B, white arrows; the characteristic metal-on-metal articulation can be seen).

The IDE multicentered clinical trial that was used to validate the safety and efficacy of Simplify was nonrandomized; its control arm was a historical cohort originally used in the RCT of its predicate metal-on-metal device, Kineflex/C. Note that the latter trial was characterized by a low 5-year follow-up rate (62.4% for ACDF), even though the 2-year equivalent was acceptable (86.5% for ACDF).[50,51] The device has completed an FDA IDE clinical trial for 2-level CTDR, also using a nonrandomized, Kineflex/C control ACDF cohort. The results of these clinical trials have been published, so far, only in the form of a 1-arm feasibility study, without performing statistical comparison with the historical ACDF cohort.[52,53] Nevertheless, the 2-year outcomes seem reassuring (mean NDI score decreased from 61.9 preoperatively to 14.8 at the 2-year follow-up; $P<.01$).

COMPARISON AMONG DEVICES
MRI Compatibility

MRI is the gold-standard imaging for degenerative disease of the spine. Most of the patients undergoing CTDR have previously been diagnosed with cervical disc herniation or spondylosis using an MRI scan. Having high-quality imaging without distortions from the metallic parts of the artificial discs during the early and late postoperative period is of paramount clinical significance. At this point, it is critical to mention that all of these devices are safe in MRI scanners of 1.5 to 3.0 T; the implantation of none of the FDA-approved artificial discs is a contraindication for MRI scanning. The degree to which each artificial disc affects the quality of imaging and the size of artifact it creates is discussed here.

In general, titanium alloy implants are considered more MRI friendly than CoCrMo alloy implants, allowing better visualization of adjacent soft tissues, such as nerves.[54] Some of the FDA-approved devices were implanted one after the other in the same cadaver and an analysis of the MRI image distortion per device was performed.[55] PRESTIGE ST, made of stainless steel, was associated with the widest artifact, distorting both index and adjacent-level image. The rule of thumb that titanium is more MRI compatible than CoCrMo was confirmed in this study, too. PRODISC-C, made of CoCrMo, produced a larger artifact than its titanium counterparts, BRYAN and PRESTIGE LP. The practical difference between the 2 metals was that the CoCrMo disc partially distorted the index level, whereas titanium discs allowed its full visualization.

Another study[56–59] evaluated images from 5 patients with each of the following devices: BRYAN, PRESTIGE LP, PRODISC-C, and PCM. The first 2 devices were again shown to correlate statistically significantly with better imaging quality than their CoCrMo homologues, with small distortion compared with the preoperative films. Both aforementioned studies used a 1.5-T MRI scanner. The Simplify disc, with its radiolucent PEEK endplates and ceramic core, has biomaterials that result in even lower image distortion than titanium-based discs.

Adjacent segment disease

There is a common pattern among the clinical trials that investigated adjacent-level degeneration in CTDR[29,60]: the rate of ASD is found to be significantly decreased at the immediately superior level, which is not the case for the immediately inferior one. This finding was partially shown in a study by Jung and colleagues,[63] who designed a biomechanical model to measure facet loading while in extension at the index and adjacent levels, in CTDR and nonoperated cervical spines.[61] At the superior level, the facet load of the CTDR model was found to be significantly decreased compared with the nonoperated cervical spine, whereas the opposite was true for the inferior and the index levels. However, facet degeneration at the index level is a contraindication to CTDR.

Nonetheless, this parameter encompasses the second pillar of inspiration of CTDR: a lower rate of ASD because of lower strain at adjacent levels. There is widespread skepticism on whether this has actually been shown, caused by major limitations in studies supporting this hypothesis, such as short follow-up periods, heterogeneity in criteria used to define ASD, variability in routine postoperative imaging protocols, and, to a small degree, imaging inaccuracies caused by hardware artifacts.[62,63] The rate of reported ASD at 1 to 3 years' follow-up has been shown to be approximately 14%, with PRODISC-C scoring higher than PRESTIGE LP, Mobi-C, and BRYAN.[64,65]

More objective evidence in support of this hypothesis is the rate of reoperations caused by ASD. Two meta-analyses have shown superiority of CTDR compared with ACDF.[66,67] However, both of these reports are limited by a maximum follow-up of 5 years. The young population undergoing CTDR combined with the slow natural course of the degenerative disease underlines the need for studies with better long-term follow-up rates to further elucidate an accurate comparison with its traditional gold-standard counterpart.

SUMMARY

CTDR is established as a viable alternative to ACDF in select patients with 1-level and 2-level cervical disorder resulting in radiculopathy.[68] Nine devices have been approved by the FDA for single-level CTDR, 2 of which have also been approved for 2-level CTDR.

CLINICS CARE POINTS

- CTDR is noninferior to ACDF in terms of overall success.
- There is no verdict, so far, as to whether CTDR is less likely than ACDF to be complicated by ASD.

DISCLOSURE

None of the authors have any conflict of interest or any other financial disclosures to report.

REFERENCES

1. Center for Devices & Radiological Health. Premarket approval (PMA) 2019. Available at: https://www.fda.gov/medical-devices/premarket-submissions/premarket-approval-pma. Accessed November 17, 2020.
2. CTCAE Files. Available at: https://evs.nci.nih.gov/ftp1/CTCAE/About.html. Accessed November 17, 2020.
3. Radcliff K, Coric D, Albert T. Five-year clinical results of cervical total disc replacement compared with anterior discectomy and fusion for treatment of 2-level symptomatic degenerative disc disease: a prospective, randomized, controlled, multicenter investigational device exemption clinical trial. J Neurosurg Spine 2016;25(2):213–24.
4. Vaccaro A, Beutler W, Peppelman W, et al. Clinical outcomes with selectively constrained SECURE-C cervical disc arthroplasty: two-year results from a prospective, randomized, controlled, multicenter investigational device exemption study. Spine (Phila Pa 1976) 2013;38(26):2227–39.
5. Premarket Approval (PMA) - PRESTIGE CERVICAL DISC SYSTEM. Available at: https://www.accessdata.fda.gov/scripts/cdrh/cfdocs/cfpma/pma.cfm?id=P060018. Accessed November 17, 2020.
6. Mummaneni PV, Burkus JK, Haid RW, et al. Clinical and radiographic analysis of cervical disc arthroplasty compared with allograft fusion: a randomized controlled clinical trial. J Neurosurg Spine 2007;6(3):198–209.
7. Staudt MD, Das K, Duggal N. Does design matter? Cervical disc replacements under review. Neurosurg Rev 2018;41(2):399–407.
8. Bertagnoli R, Yue JJ, Pfeiffer F, et al. Early results after ProDisc-C cervical disc replacement. J Neurosurg Spine 2005;2(4):403–10.
9. Murrey D, Janssen M, Delamarter R, et al. Results of the prospective, randomized, controlled multicenter Food and Drug Administration investigational device exemption study of the ProDisc-C total disc replacement versus anterior discectomy and fusion for the treatment of 1-level symptomatic cervical disc disease. Spine J 2009;9(4):275–86.
10. Delamarter RB, Zigler J. Five-year reoperation rates, cervical total disc replacement versus fusion, results of a prospective randomized clinical trial. Spine (Phila Pa 1976) 2013;38(9):711–7.
11. Janssen ME, Zigler JE, Spivak JM, et al. ProDisc-C Total Disc Replacement Versus Anterior Cervical Discectomy and Fusion for Single-Level Symptomatic Cervical Disc Disease: Seven-Year Follow-up of the Prospective Randomized U.S. Food and Drug Administration Investigational Device Exemption Study. J Bone Joint Surg Am 2015;97(21):1738–47.
12. Radcliff K, Lerner J, Yang C, et al. Seven-year cost-effectiveness of ProDisc-C total disc replacement: results from investigational device exemption and post-approval studies. J Neurosurg Spine 2016;24(5):760–8.
13. Premarket Approval (PMA) - PRODISC TM-C TOTAL DISC REPLACEMENT. Available at: https://www.accessdata.fda.gov/scripts/cdrh/cfdocs/cfpma/pma.cfm?id=P070001. Accessed November 17, 2020.
14. Premarket Approval (PMA) - BRYAN CERVICAL DISC PROSTHESIS. Available at: https://www.accessdata.fda.gov/scripts/cdrh/cfdocs/cfpma/pma.cfm?id=P060023. Accessed November 17, 2020.
15. Bryan VE Jr. Cervical motion segment replacement. Eur Spine J 2002;11(Suppl 2):S92–7.
16. Goffin J, Casey A, Kehr P, et al. Preliminary clinical experience with the Bryan Cervical Disc Prosthesis. Neurosurgery 2002;51(3):840–7.
17. Heller JG, Sasso RC, Papadopoulos SM, et al. Comparison of BRYAN cervical disc arthroplasty with anterior cervical decompression and fusion: clinical and radiographic results of a randomized, controlled, clinical trial. Spine (Phila Pa 1976) 2009;34(2):101–7.
18. Lavelle WF, Riew KD, Levi AD, et al. Ten-year Outcomes of Cervical Disc Replacement With the BRYAN Cervical Disc: Results From a Prospective, Randomized, Controlled Clinical Trial. Spine (Phila Pa 1976) 2019;44(9):601–8.

19. Cheng L, Nie L, Zhang L, et al. Fusion versus Bryan Cervical Disc in two-level cervical disc disease: a prospective, randomised study. Int Orthop 2009; 33(5):1347–51.

20. Pointillart V, Castelain JE, Coudert P, et al. Outcomes of the Bryan cervical disc replacement: fifteen year follow-up. Int Orthop 2018;42(4):851–7.

21. Fay LY, Huang WC, Tsai TY, et al. Differences between arthroplasty and anterior cervical fusion in two-level cervical degenerative disc disease. Eur Spine J 2014;23(3):627–34.

22. Premarket Approval (PMA) - SECURE-C ARTIFICIAL CERVICAL DISC. Available at: https://www.accessdata.fda.gov/scripts/cdrh/cfdocs/cfpma/pma.cfm?id=P100003. Accessed November 17, 2020.

23. Vaccaro A, Beutler W, Peppelman W, et al. Long-Term Clinical Experience with Selectively Constrained SECURE-C Cervical Artificial Disc for 1-Level Cervical Disc Disease: Results from Seven-Year Follow-Up of a Prospective, Randomized, Controlled Investigational Device Exemption Clinical Trial. Int J Spine Surg 2018;12(3):377–87.

24. Pimenta L, McAfee PC, Cappuccino A, et al. Clinical experience with the new artificial cervical PCM (Cervitech) disc. Spine J 2004;4(6 Suppl):315S–21S.

25. Pimenta L, McAfee PC, Cappuccino A, et al. Superiority of multilevel cervical arthroplasty outcomes versus single-level outcomes: 229 consecutive PCM prostheses. Spine (Phila Pa 1976) 2007; 32(12):1337–44.

26. Odom GL, Finney W, Woodhall B. Cervical disk lesions. J Am Med Assoc 1958;166(1):23–8.

27. Phillips FM, Lee JY, Geisler FH, et al. A prospective, randomized, controlled clinical investigation comparing PCM cervical disc arthroplasty with anterior cervical discectomy and fusion. 2-year results from the US FDA IDE clinical trial. Spine (Phila Pa 1976) 2013;38(15):E907–18.

28. Premarket Approval (PMA) - NUVASIVE PCM CERVICAL DISC SYSTEM. Available at: https://www.accessdata.fda.gov/scripts/cdrh/cfdocs/cfpma/pma.cfm?id=P100012. Accessed November 17, 2020.

29. Phillips FM, Geisler FH, Gilder KM, et al. Long-term Outcomes of the US FDA IDE Prospective, Randomized Controlled Clinical Trial Comparing PCM Cervical Disc Arthroplasty With Anterior Cervical Discectomy and Fusion. Spine (Phila Pa 1976) 2015;40(10):674–83.

30. Hisey MS, Bae HW, Davis R, et al. Multi-center, prospective, randomized, controlled investigational device exemption clinical trial comparing Mobi-C Cervical Artificial Disc to anterior discectomy and fusion in the treatment of symptomatic degenerative disc disease in the cervical spine. Int J Spine Surg 2014;8:7.

31. Beaurain J, Bernard P, Dufour T, et al. Intermediate clinical and radiological results of cervical TDR (Mobi-C) with up to 2 years of follow-up. Eur Spine J 2009;18(6):841–50.

32. Davis RJ, Kim KD, Hisey MS, et al. Cervical total disc replacement with the Mobi-C cervical artificial disc compared with anterior discectomy and fusion for treatment of 2-level symptomatic degenerative disc disease: a prospective, randomized, controlled multicenter clinical trial. J Neurosurg Spine 2013; 19(5):532–45.

33. Radcliff KE, Davis RJ, Hoffman GA, et al. Seven-Year Clinical Results of Cervical Total Disc Replacement Compared with Anterior Discectomy and Fusion for Treatment of Two-Level Symptomatic Degenerative Disc Disease: A Prospective, Randomized, Controlled, Multicenter FDA Clinical Trial. Spine J 2016;16(10):S204.

34. Premarket Approval (PMA) - MOBI-C CERVICAL DISC PROSTHESIS (ONE-LEVEL INDICATION). Available at: https://www.accessdata.fda.gov/scripts/cdrh/cfdocs/cfpma/pma.cfm?id=P110002. Accessed November 17, 2020.

35. Premarket Approval (PMA) - MOBI-C CERVICAL DISC PROSTHESIS (TWO-LEVEL INDICATION). Available at: https://www.accessdata.fda.gov/scripts/cdrh/cfdocs/cfpma/pma.cfm?id=P110009. Accessed November 17, 2020.

36. Ament JD, Yang Z, Nunley P, et al. Cost Utility Analysis of the Cervical Artificial Disc vs Fusion for the Treatment of 2-Level Symptomatic Degenerative Disc Disease: 5-Year Follow-up. Neurosurgery 2016;79(1):135–45.

37. Premarket Approval (PMA) - PRESTIGE LP CERVICAL DISC. Available at: https://www.accessdata.fda.gov/scripts/cdrh/cfdocs/cfpma/pma.cfm?%20id=P090029. Accessed November 17, 2020.

38. Gornet MF, Lanman TH, Burkus JK, et al. Cervical disc arthroplasty with the Prestige LP disc versus anterior cervical discectomy and fusion, at 2 levels: results of a prospective, multicenter randomized controlled clinical trial at 24 months. J Neurosurg Spine 2017;26(6):653–67.

39. Lanman TH, Burkus JK, Dryer RG, et al. Long-term clinical and radiographic outcomes of the Prestige LP artificial cervical disc replacement at 2 levels: results from a prospective randomized controlled clinical trial. J Neurosurg Spine 2017;27(1):7–19.

40. McAnany SJ, Merrill RK, Overley SC, et al. Investigating the 7-Year Cost-Effectiveness of Single-Level Cervical Disc Replacement Compared to Anterior Cervical Discectomy and Fusion. Glob Spine J 2018;8(1):32–9.

41. Merrill RK, McAnany SJ, Albert TJ, et al. Is Two-level Cervical Disc Replacement More Cost-effective Than Anterior Cervical Discectomy and Fusion at 7 Years? Spine (Phila Pa 1976) 2018;43(9):610–6.

42. Kim JS, Dowdell J, Cheung ZB, et al. The Seven-Year Cost-Effectiveness of Anterior Cervical Discectomy and Fusion Versus Cervical Disc Arthroplasty: A Markov Analysis. Spine (Phila Pa 1976) 2018; 43(22):1543–51.

43. Carreon LY, Anderson PA, Traynelis VC, et al. Cost-effectiveness of single-level anterior cervical discectomy and fusion five years after surgery. Spine (Phila Pa 1976) 2013;38(6):471–5.

44. Premarket Approval (PMA) - PRESTIGE LP(TM) CERVICAL DISC. Available at: https://www.accessdata.fda.gov/scripts/cdrh/cfdocs/cfpma/pma.cfm?ID=353100. Accessed November 17, 2020.

45. Reyes-Sanchez A, Miramontes V, Olivarez LM, et al. Initial clinical experience with a next-generation artificial disc for the treatment of symptomatic degenerative cervical radiculopathy. SAS J 2010;4(1):9–15.

46. Thomas S, Willems K, Van den Daelen L, et al. The M6-C Cervical Disk Prosthesis: First Clinical Experience in 33 Patients. Clin Spine Surg 2016;29(4): E182–7.

47. Premarket Approval (PMA) - M6-C Artificial Cervical Disc. Available at: https://www.accessdata.fda.gov/scripts/cdrh/cfdocs/cfpma/pma.cfm?id=P170036. Accessed November 17, 2020.

48. Phillips FM, Coric D, Sasso R, et al. Prospective, multicenter clinical trial comparing M6-C compressible six degrees of freedom cervical disc with anterior cervical discectomy and fusion for the treatment of single-level degenerative cervical radiculopathy: 2-year results of an FDA investigational device exemption study. Spine J 2021;21(2):239–52.

49. Center for Devices & Radiological Health. Simplify Cervical Artificial Disc - P200022. Available at: https://www.fda.gov/medical-devices/recently-approved-devices/simplify-cervical-artificial-disc-p200022. Accessed November 17, 2020.

50. Coric D, Nunley PD, Guyer RD, et al. Prospective, randomized, multicenter study of cervical arthroplasty: 269 patients from the Kineflex|C artificial disc investigational device exemption study with a minimum 2-year follow-up: clinical article. J Neurosurg Spine 2011;15(4):348–58.

51. Coric D, Guyer RD, Nunley PD, et al. Prospective, randomized multicenter study of cervical arthroplasty versus anterior cervical discectomy and fusion: 5-year results with a metal-on-metal artificial disc. J Neurosurg Spine 2018;28(3):252–61.

52. Coric D, Guyer RD, Carmody CN, et al, Cervical Disc Replacement Using a PEEK-on-Ceramic Implant: Prospective Data from Seven Sites Participating in an FDA IDE Trial for Single-level Surgery [abstract]. In: North American Spine Society Meeting; 2020 Oct 9; Virtual Conference. The Spine J; 2020. Abstract no. 161.

53. Guyer RD, Nunley PD, Strenge KB, et al. 162. Two-level cervical disc replacement using a PEEK-on-ceramic device: prospective outcome data from an FDA IDE trial. Spine J 2020;20:S80–1.

54. Rupp R, Ebraheim NA, Savolaine ER, et al. Magnetic Resonance Imaging Evaluation of the Spine With Metal Implants|General Safety and Superior Imaging With Titanium. Spine 1993;18(3): 279–385.

55. Fayyazi AH, Taormina J, Svach D, et al. Assessment of Magnetic Resonance Imaging Artifact Following Cervical Total Disc Arthroplasty. Int J Spine Surg 2015;9:30.

56. Sekhon LH, Duggal N, Lynch JJ, et al. Magnetic resonance imaging clarity of the Bryan, Prodisc-C, Prestige LP, and PCM cervical arthroplasty devices. Spine (Phila Pa 1976) 2007;32(6):673–80.

57. McAfee PC, Cunningham BW, Devine J, et al. Classification of heterotopic ossification (HO) in artificial disk replacement. J Spinal Disord Tech 2003;16(4): 384–9.

58. Nunley PD, Cavanaugh DA, Kerr EJ, et al. Heterotopic Ossification After Cervical Total Disc Replacement at 7 Years-Prevalence, Progression, Clinical Implications, and Risk Factors. Int J Spine Surg 2018;12(3):352–61.

59. Yi S, Kim KN, Yang MS, et al. Difference in occurrence of heterotopic ossification according to prosthesis type in the cervical artificial disc replacement. Spine (Phila Pa 1976) 2010;35(16): 1556–61.

60. Wahood W, Yolcu YU, Kerezoudis P, et al. Artificial Discs in Cervical Disc Replacement: A Meta-Analysis for Comparison of Long-Term Outcomes. World Neurosurg 2020;134:598.e5.

61. Virk S, Phillips F, Khan S, et al. A cross-sectional analysis of 1347 complications for cervical disc replacements from medical device reports maintained by the United States Food and Drug Administration. Spine J 2020. https://doi.org/10.1016/j.spinee.2020.09.005.

62. Zhai S, Li A, Li X, et al. Total disc replacement compared with fusion for cervical degenerative disc disease: A systematic review of overlapping meta-analyses. Medicine 2020;99:e20143.

63. Jung T-G, Woo S-H, Park K-M, et al. Biomechanical behavior of two different cervical total disc replacement designs in relation of concavity of articular surfaces: ProDisc-C® vs. Prestige-LP®. Int J Precis Eng Manuf 2013;14(5):819–24.

64. Bartels RHMA, Donk R, Verbeek ALM. No justification for cervical disk prostheses in clinical practice: a meta-analysis of randomized controlled trials. Neurosurgery 2010;66:1153–60 [discussion: 1160].

65. Jawahar A, Cavanaugh DA, Kerr EJ, et al. Total disc arthroplasty does not affect the incidence of

adjacent segment degeneration in cervical spine: results of 93 patients in three prospective randomized clinical trials. Spine J 2010;10(12):1043–8.

66. Upadhyaya CD, Wu JC, Trost G, et al. Analysis of the three United States Food and Drug Administration investigational device exemption cervical arthroplasty trials. J Neurosurg Spine 2012;16(3): 216–28.

67. Zhang Y, Liang C, Tao Y, et al. Cervical total disc replacement is superior to anterior cervical decompression and fusion: a meta-analysis of prospective randomized controlled trials. PLoS One 2015;10(3): e0117826.

68. Coric D, Mummaneni PV, Traynelis V, et al. Introduction: Cervical arthroplasty. Neurosurg Focus 2017; 42(2):E1.

Cervical Total Disc Replacement: Expanded Indications

Óscar L. Alves, MD[a,b],*

KEYWORDS

- Multilevel cervical total disc replacement • 3- or 4-level cervical disc arthroplasty
- Cervical artificial disc • Cervical motion preservation • Off-label spine surgery • ACDF
- Cervical spondylotic myelopathy • Degenerative disc disease

KEY POINTS

- As an alternative to fusion surgery, cTDR represents an opportunity window to treat earlier younger patients with moderate forms of multilevel myelopathy achieving an MCID in clinical outcomes.
- Hybrid constructs constitute a valid option for patients with different stages of spondylosis progression. cTDR may be used in less spondylotic levels or in those expected to have a higher range of motion.
- Regarding the surgical technique in multilevel cTDR, it is crucial to rely both on direct decompression and proper device insertion to achieve the best biokinematic outcomes that will translate in superior clinical outcomes.
- The beneficial effect of cTDR on cervical spine alignment is not inferior to ACDF, as motion preservation allows for proper alignment compensations. This combination is favorable for multilevel cTDR patients.
- The rate of adjacent segment disease and adjacent segment reoperation is lower in multilevel patients who underwent cTDR than ACDF. cTDR superiority increases over time.

INTRODUCTION

Anterior cervical discectomy and fusion (ACDF) is traditionally regarded as the gold standard treatment for either single-level or multilevel compressive cervical disc disease. However, over the last 15 years, several US Federal Drug Administration (FDA) Investigational Device Exemption (IDE) Prospective Randomized Controlled (PRC) trials with different devices, as well as systematic reviews and meta-analysis, furnished robust level 1 and 2 data supporting the use of 1- and 2-level cervical total disc replacement (cTDR) as a valid clinical alternative to ACDF.[1–4] Significantly, long-term (>5 years) follow-up enhances the difference in clinical outcomes between cTDR and ACDF, and results for 2-level cTDR are even more consistent than those for a single level.[1,5]

In comparison to Europe and Asia, there is a biased resistance in North America to consent with multilevel cTDR. The lack of compliance is multifactorial in nature; it relates to lack of FDA approval, to codification and reimbursement issues, to implant costs, to longer and more technically demanding surgeries, and to heterotopic ossification (HO).[6,7] However, given that motion elimination at multiple levels causes an unquestionably negative impact on patients' quality of

[a] Hospital Lusíadas Porto; [b] Centro Hospitalar de Gaia/Espinho, Rua Cónego Ferreira Pinto, 191, 4050-256 Porto, Portugal
* Centro Hospitalar de Gaia/Espinho, Rua Cónego Ferreira Pinto, 191, 4050-256 Porto, Portugal.
E-mail address: oscar.l.alves@gmail.com

Neurosurg Clin N Am 32 (2021) 437–448
https://doi.org/10.1016/j.nec.2021.05.002
1042-3680/21/© 2021 Elsevier Inc. All rights reserved.

life, as cervical spine is designed for motion, it would be expected that in more than 2-level degenerative disc disease (DDD), cTDR would have a widespread appeal. The potential growth of this technique is evident in the context of rising incidence of multilevel disc disease among younger patients who will poorly tolerate multilevel fusion[8] (**Fig. 1**).

Multiple level ACDF constructs cause a substantial biomechanical fingerprint on adjacent natural levels, accelerating adjacent segment disease (ASD) to a rate of 25% at 10 years.[9] Owing to the progressive increase in stiffness, multilevel fusion opposed to a single-level fusion constructs magnify the increase of adjacent segment hypermobility.[10] Not surprisingly, after multilevel ACDF,

the incidence of hardware failure and complications is incremental with the number of operated levels.[11] A systematic review by Jiang and colleagues reported pseudarthrosis rates of 37.3% for 3-level and 33.3% for 4-level procedures.[12] Despite these noteworthy drawbacks associated with ACDF, 3- and 4-level cTDR has never gained a real widespread acceptance, likely because of a lack of firm evidence basis.[13] Most of the reports, including a small number of patients, emerged from Out of United States (OUS) practice. To date, no US IDE study has included patients with cervical DDD at more than 2-levels.

As an existing FDA recommendation allows up to 2-levels cTDR with selected disc prosthesis, the multilevel concept used in this article relates

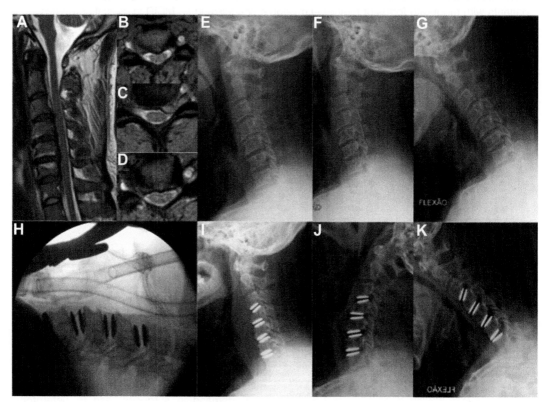

Fig. 1. cTDR in a 4-level degenerative disc disease case. A 45-year-old male presenting with neck pain (VAS 5), multiradicular arm pain (VAS 8) bilateral hand paresthesia, left dysesthesia C6 and C7 with an mJoA = 13. The patient became asymptomatic, except for sporadic neck pain (VAS 2), and fully recovered fine motor skills and sensory deficits (A): sagittal T2-weighted MRI showing spinal cord compression at disc level from C3-7; (B–D): axial T2-weighted MRI confirming spinal cord and nerve roots compression C4-5, C5-6 and C6-7; (E–G): lateral dynamic cervical radiographs exhibiting a suboptimal global ROM and ruling out major instability and spondylosis; (H): intra-operative lateral x-ray confirming adequate neural elements decompression, proper implant placement and sagittal alignment. (I–K): 3-year postoperative lateral dynamic cervical radiographs showing proper mobility of the disc prosthesis, improvement of sagittal balance parameters on neutral view and absence of heterotopic calcification. C2-7 and C0-2 angles changed from 1.5° to 6.8° and from 52.3° to 38.5°, respectively, global ROM improved from 34.2° to 58.9°, SVA increased slightly from 34.8 mm to 41.1 mm, and T1 slope changed from 33.2° to 25.6°. mJoA, modified Japanese Orthopedic Association scale for myelopathy; ROM, range of motion; SVA, sagittal vertical alignment; VAS, visual analogue scale.

to 3- or 4-level cervical disc disease as synonymous with "expanded" indications. In this article, a quest for evidence for the use of cTDR, alone or adjacent to fusion, in 3- and 4-level disc disease is undertaken.

Indications and Contraindications for more than 2-Level Cervical Total Disc Replacement

An expanded indication to 3- and 4-level cTDR can be performed in patients with milder or moderate forms of multilevel radiculopathy/myelopathy. Typically, these are younger patients with greater life expectancy, not affected by osteoporosis, as well as with minimal facet joint degeneration, but presenting with substantial disease burden when assessed using quality-of-life scales. If their preoperative baseline modified Japanese Orthopedic Association scale for myelopathy (mJOA) scores are higher or if their symptom duration is shorter, surgery will produce a dramatic improvement in those measures at 2-year follow-up.[14] Multilevel cTDR may represent a window of opportunity to treat earlier patients with moderate forms of myelopathy achieving Minimal Clinically Important Difference (MCID) on clinical outcome scales (see **Fig. 1**).

Advanced disc degenerative Modic changes (>grade 2), facet degeneration related to axial neck pain, as well as a circumferential cord compression with a section around the cord<6 mm are contraindications for multilevel cTDR. In 37 patients with 3-level myelopathy from congenital spinal stenosis, Chang PY and colleagues found that motion preservation (hybrid 2-level cTDR with 1-level ACDF) yielded similar long-term outcomes as motion elimination (3-level ACDF).[15] Inclusion criteria for enrollment in this study were age (<50 years) and cervical canal stenosis as defined by a Pavlov ratio ≤ 0.82. However, as excessive motion may contribute to the worsening of myelopathy, motion preservation is questionable in moderate to severe forms of cervical myelopathy.

The preoperative CT scan is useful for the detection of facet arthropathy, calcified disc, osteophytes, ossification of the posterior longitudinal ligament (OPLL). In a study of 15 patients with severe 3-level cervical myelopathy from OPLL, Chang and colleagues found that hybrid surgery with cTDR combined with 1-level anterior cervical corpectomy resulted in improvement in Neck Disability Index (NDI), mJOA, and preserved range of motion (ROM) across the cTDR level at 12 months postoperatively.[16] But, OPLL, other than the localized type behind the disc, is a contraindication for cervical arthroplasty.

Both anteroposterior and lateral cervical radiographs can provide useful information regarding the eligibility for multilevel cTDR. Pre-existing cervical kyphotic deformity greater than 15°, severe ankylosis, and spondylosis are considered contraindications for cervical arthroplasty. On the dynamic lateral radiographs, the restriction to motion due to facet joint arthrosis or the presence of instability (>3 mm translation/subluxation), both disqualify for cTDR. Whenever translational instability is present in multilevel disease, nonconstrained implants are not recommended because they are placed under a biomechanical stress beyond their capacity to maintain stability. In multilevel DDD, each individual level considered for cTDR needs to be carefully scrutinized to identify the aforementioned contraindications, as summarized in **Box 1**.

Surgical Technique for Multilevel Cervical Total Disc Replacement

When performing 3- or 4-level cTDR, a standard anterior cervical approach is carried out while the patient is on supine position. Depending on the depth of the cervical spine to the surface, a horizontal or vertical skin incision is done with similar cosmetic results. It is recommended to avoid hyperextension of the neck to prevent intraoperative neural damage and to avoid implant oversize that relates to the late occurrence of subsidence and segmental kyphosis. Therefore, a perfect neck positioning should be assessed by lateral fluoroscopy.

Assuring proper spinal cord and nerve root decompression is the primary goal of cTDR, which

---

Box 1
Exclusion criteria for cTDR in multilevel cervical degenerative disc disease

Cervical radiographs: kyphotic deformity greater than 15°, spondylosis with decreased disc height

Dynamic cervical radiographs: segmental motion restriction due to fused facets, instability (>3 mm translation/subluxation

CT: large osteophytes, OPLL, ankylosis, facet arthropathy

MRI: significant facet joint degeneration, Modic changes >2, SAC<6 mm

DEXA Scan: significant osteoporosis (T-score<1.5)

Abbreviations: DEXA scan, bone density scan; SAC, section around the cord.

is not different from ACDF. However, a major discrepancy in terms of the extent of foraminal decompression exists between ACDF and cTDR. Foraminal decompression needs to be exhaustive with cTDR, as the surgeon cannot rely only in indirect decompression offered by the implant height. At the index segment, residual bony foraminal stenosis may result in recurrent radiculopathy. Direct decompression is a crucial concept in cTDR surgical technique.

Using a 4-mm burr, a "shaving" drilling technique with extra care to avoid end-plate damage can be used to reformat a disc space to fit the disc prosthesis. This is of utmost importance in more spondylotic levels, as it is often the case in multilevel disc disease. A perfect, flat, and smooth endplate preparation helps primary stability of parallel end plates cervical disc prosthesis (see **Fig. 1**). Posterior longitudinal ligament removal is recommended for several reasons: to remove extruded disc material posterior to the ligament and osteophytes, passing with the 2-mm punch under the ligament, and to avoid a scaffold for later posterior HO. Removal of posterior ligament has a negligible impact on index segment postoperative hypermobility as it increases rotation by only 0.5°.[17] Motion segment stiffness loss after PLL resection can be compensated by a TDR design that can provide graded resistance to angular motion.

At the end of the decompression when facing the decision to insert or not a cTDR device, the intraoperative mobility between two vertebral bodies can be assessed through a simple leverage maneuver with the suction cannula. Because of concerns with the reduced bone density in multilevel patients, vertebral body pins are placed only at the moment of the disc prosthesis insertion when external cervical spine traction is not enough to open a couple of millimeters of the disc space.

Contrary to cage insertion to promote fusion in ACDF, special care is recommended to ensure a proper placement of the implant in cTDR, both in the sagittal plane as well as in the coronal plane, using the uncus as reference on an anteroposterior fluoroscopy. In multilevel patients, accurate placement and alignment is crucial for a superior biomechanical performance of the cervical disc prosthesis that relates with better outcomes and complication avoidance, especially HO.

In multilevel cases, surgical decompression is generally started from the caudal to the cephalad levels except in cases of frank cord compression which is typically addressed first. The insertion of cervical disc prosthesis progresses, similarly, in a caudal to cephalad fashion. Although there is no literature demonstrating the superiority of one implant over the other in multilevel disease, it is advised to avoid using implants with a prominent keel, fin, or screws to avoid vertebral body fracture, subsidence, or loss of anterior body height in the long term. Cervical disc prosthesis with the proper height, commonly 6-mm high or less in most patients, and the largest footprint possible should be chosen to avoid complications as subsidence, migration, heterotopic calcification, or absence of segmental motion by splaying the facet joints.

Current Evidence for Multilevel Cervical Total Disc Replacement

Clinical outcomes

Concerning 3- and 4-level, Laratta and colleagues reported at 24-month reductions of 26.1% in NDI, 33.4% in neck pain, and 50.4% in arm pain in comparison with intermediate 12-month follow-up for ACDF.[11] Pimenta and colleagues found favorable outcomes in a subgroup of cTDR (12 patients with 3-level and 4 with 4-level) at 3-year follow-up.[18] In Asia, 3-level cTDR data through 10 years showed good results but high rates of HO.[19] Comparing a matched cohort of 50 patients with 3-level cTDR versus ACDF with a 24-month follow-up, Chang and colleagues concluded that clinical outcomes (neck visual analogue score [nVAS], arm visual analogue score [aVAS], NDI, mJOA) improved for both groups when compared with the patients' preoperative condition.[20] In a literature review that included 3 prospective randomized studies and several retrospective studies (n = 1554, of which 947 were multilevel including cohorts with 3- and 4-level cTDR), Joaquim and Riew added evidence in favor of cTDR for multilevel disc disease.[21] In 4 out of 5, cTDR either showed significant clinical superiority over ACDF or a trend in that direction.

The analysis of cTDR cohorts found no major significant differences when increasing the number of implants in individual patients. Huppert and colleagues at 2-year follow-up found a similar degree of improvement from baseline for clinical outcomes (NDI, nVAS, aVAS, Short Form Health Survey (SF-36) quality of life score, return to work, satisfaction and success rates) and in complications and reoperation rates between single (n = 175 patients, n = 175 implants) and multilevel (n = 56 patients, n = 118 implants) cTDR.[22] However, their study included only 4 patients treated at 3-level and 1 patient treated at 4-level cTDR. Gornet and colleagues in a study enrolling 3-level (n = 116) and 4-level (n = 23) patients undergoing cTDR showed that patients-reported-outcomes scores improved significantly at all postoperative intervals $(P < .001)$.[23] Patient satisfaction exceeded 88% seven years after surgery. They concluded that 3- and 4-level cTDR can be performed safely and effectively in appropriately selected patients with multilevel disease.[23] Subgroup analysis from Reinas and colleagues data concerning pure multilevel cTDR (n = 32 patients) showed that for 3- and 4-level groups, both nVAS and aVAS scores improved significantly similar to 2-level cTDR patients,[24] as shown in **Table 1**. Remarkably, a 100% favorable outcome by Odom's criteria was shown compared with 85.7% in 2-level cTDR patients. Despite the low evidence level and low enrollment, it can be suggested that adding cTDR devices to the final construct does not limit the clinical benefit offered by single-level cTDR. Moreover, there is a trend for a superior benefit in 3- and 4-level patients. None of the publications on 3- and 4-level cTDR patients report an increase in complication rate in comparison to 1- and 2-level TDR, or multilevel ACDF.

Radiological Outcomes

Motion preservation at the index level is the primary radiological outcome that differentiates cTDR from ADCF. Retaining multilevel disc mobility is of paramount importance to reach favorable clinical outcomes, especially in 3- and 4-level disc disease. In a study with mean follow-up of 44.5 months (19–70 months), Reinas and colleagues found for the index level ROM a gain in mobility of $1.3 \pm 8.1°$ per level in 3- and 4-level groups, while 2-level cTDR gained $1.1 \pm 4.7°$[24] (see **Table 1**). Chang and colleagues also reported

a mean ROM increase of approximately 3.4° (3-level sum) after the 3-level surgery $(P = .001)$.[20] From a biokinematic point of view, the capacity of each implant to display appropriate mobility does not appear to be compromised by assembling more cervical disc prostheses in a single patient. Compared with baseline global ROM, a statistically significant increase of $7.2 \pm 11.7°$ $(P = .07)$ in 3- or 4-level was observed, whereas for 2-level patients, an increment was visible but not significant $(1.6 \pm 9.4°; P = .44)$.[24] Therefore, it may be much more clinically relevant and meaningful to offer cTDR to 3- and 4-level disc disease patients than to 2-level patients in whom adjacent natural levels can individually compensate for the loss of mobility observed with fusion. Moreover, the significant increase in global ROM in 3- and 4-level patients $(7.2 \pm 11.7°)$ is in striking contrast with the complete loss of mobility created by 3- and 4-level fusion surgery.

Besides ROM, quality of motion is critical for the outcome of cTDR surgery in multilevel patients as an altered center of rotation (COR) may affect negatively segmental and global ROM (Pagaimo F, Fernandes P, Xavier J, et al. New methodology to assess in-vivo quality of motion in cervical spine. In submission to Clin Biomech). Artificial discs with a mobile core having an additional degree of freedom, anterior-posterior translation, and a compressible property will allow a more "physiologic" COR that will effectively lower the mechanical load over adjacent discs.[25]

Concerning cervical spine alignment, kyphosis, and increased sagittal vertical axis (SVA) are linked

Table 1
Comparative demographics, clinical and radiological outcomes for 3- and 4-level versus 2-level cTDR, according to Reinas et al[24]

cTDR	2-Level	3- and 4-Level
Patients (n = 32)	21	11
Mean age (range), y	45 (30–63)	47 (42–58)
Index levels (n)	42	35
Mean FU (range), m	45 (30–63)	44.5 (19–70)
nVAS	7.2 ± 1.2–2.7 ± 1.5*	7.9 ± 0.5–1.5 ± 1.5*
aVAS	5.9 ± 1.9–2.1 ± 1.6*	7.1 ± 1.6–2.2 ± 1.8*
Favorable outcome (Odom's)	18/21 (85.7%)	11/11 (100%)
Mean ΔC2-7 angle (SD)	1.2 (6.36)	3.9 (8.51)
Mean Δ index angle (SD)	1.6 (5.17)	1.3 (8.51)
Mean ΔSVA (SD)	−1.3 (8.08)	−3.4 6.26)
Mean iΔROM (SD)	1.1 (4.67)	1.3 (8.08)
Mean gΔROM (SD)	1.6 (9.4)	7.2 (11.74)*
>2 y FU, Incidence HO, %	4/39 (11%)	3/35 (8.6%)

Abbreviation: FU, follow-up.

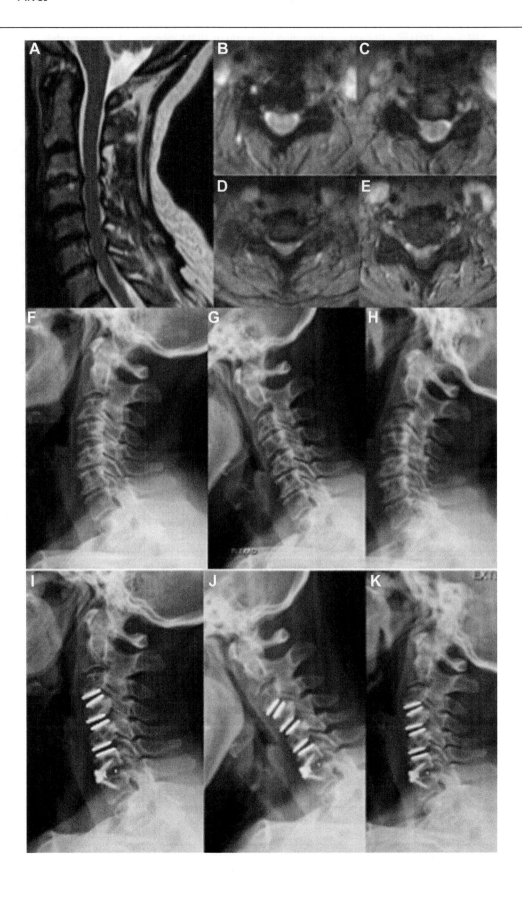

to postoperative pain, disability, and progression of myelopathy. It is, thus, crucial to demonstrate that multilevel cTDR can preserve cervical alignment. In a study on 3-level surgery, Hung and colleagues noticed that postoperative SVA was greater (no significant difference) in the TDR group (n = 20 patients) than ACDF (n = 20 patients) and hybrid surgery (n = 22 patients).[26] They concluded that TDR is not a good choice for large preoperative SVA. Reinas and associates demonstrated that 2-level and 3- to 4-level cTDR groups presented similar effects on sagittal balance with an increase in global lordosis and decrease in SVA[24] as described in **Table 1**. Multilevel cTDR may produce encouraging effects on global lordosis and SVA, which coupled with motion preservation is relevant for the overall clinical outcomes.

Current Evidence for Multilevel Hybrid Constructs

Hybrid constructs (combining in the same construct cTDR and ACDF) may represent a valid option for patients with multilevel disc disease at different stages of spondylosis progression (**Fig. 2**). From a biomechanical point of view and respecting cTDR contraindications, cTDR may be used in levels that are less spondylotic or expected to have a higher ROM (eg, C5-6 as opposed to C6-7), whereas fusion can be applied in the more spondylotic, less mobile, or high slippage levels. Significantly, cTDR placed adjacent to a fusion is subjected to a more challenging biomechanical environment than stand alone. This additional biokinematic recruitment can accommodate increased moment loads without subsidence or undue wear during the expected life of the prosthesis.[27]

Despite existing data reporting sound clinical and radiological outcomes, there have been no FDA approvals for the hybrid indication. In their meta-analysis (n = 442 patients) comparing multilevel hybrid constructs to multilevel ACDF and cTDR, Hollyer and colleagues found that NDI and VAS were similar to those of multilevel cTDR with an improvement in both global and segmental ROM and a shorter return to work than ACDF.[28] Hung and colleagues found hybrid construct superior compared with 3-level cTDR in restoring cervical lordosis and SVA.[26] By combining the best features of both fusion and motion preservation, hybrid constructs have a favorable biomechanics profile because they preserve ROM with minimal changes in COR (Pagaimo F, Fernandes P, Xavier J, et al. New methodology to assess in-vivo quality of motion in cervical spine. In submission to Clin Biomech).

A pertinent topic in progressive multiple level DDD is the surgical management of ASD next to a previous fusion (**Fig. 3**). cTDR devices were used in 12 single-level and 9 multilevel cases contiguous to prior fusions by Pimenta and colleagues with positive results.[18] Huppert and colleagues also added cTDR to earlier fusions and reported similar results.[22] According to Lu and colleagues, cTDR confers similar surgical and performance outcomes in the treatment of ASD as ACDF.[29] It is also feasible to insert a cTDR device to revise a failed fusion, but only 31 cases have been identified so far in subgroup analysis.[18,22,30]

Adjacent Segment Disease and Reoperation After Multilevel Cervical Total Disc Replacement

A key theoretic benefit of cTDR is the mitigation of ASD when compared with fusion surgery. A combination of increase in motion coupled with increased intradiscal pressure and facets load at adjacent levels may accelerate ASD after fusion. Many biomechanical studies have established that cTDR minimizes these negative kinematic effects.[31]

However, the stiffness created by fusion at the index level is only one factor in developing ASD. Another immutable factor is the natural history of the underlying cervical spondylosis. Fortunately, it seems clear that most radiological ASD has no clinical correlation and, therefore, is not equivalent to adjacent segment reoperation (ASR).

Fig. 2. Hybrid construct for 4-level degenerative disc disease, including cTDR at C3-4, C4-5, and C5-6, and ACDF at C6-7. A 69-year-old female presenting with neck and nuchal pain (VAS 6) of a burning sensation, multiradicular arm pain (VAS 7), grade 4 hand grip with myelopathic signs mJoA = 13. (A) Cervical T2-weighted MRI sagittal views showing compression from C3 to C7; (B–E) cervical T2-weighted MRI axial views showing spinal cord and nerve root compression at 4 level from C3 to C7; (F H) preoperative neutral lateral cervical radiograph denoting a balanced cervical spine with multilevel spondylosis; (I–K): 2-year postoperative dynamic, flexion and extension, lateral cervical radiographs showing a good sagittal balance, reformatting of the disc height, proper function of the cervical disc prosthesis and absence of heterotopic ossification. C2-7 and C0-2 angles changed from 34° to 22.4° and from 27.9° to 33°, respectively, global ROM decreased marginally from 33.9° to 31.2°, SVA increased from 4.3 mm to 15.8 mm, and T1 slope changed from 38.5° to 26.9°. VAS, visual analog scale.

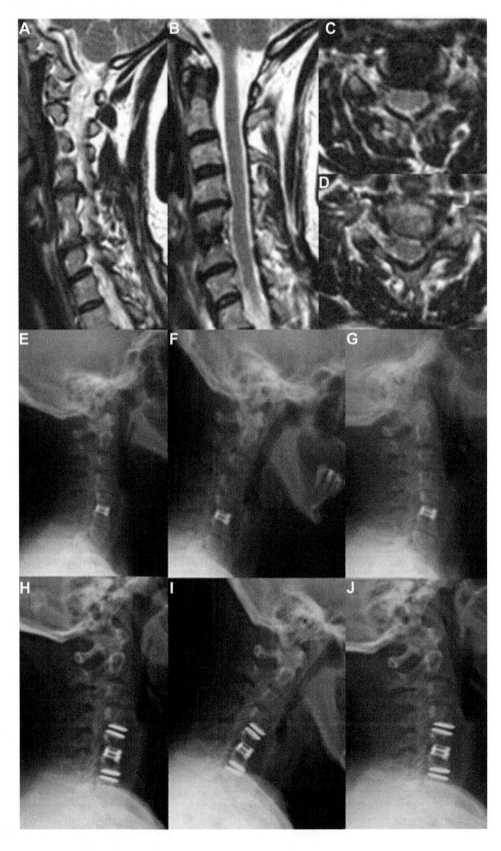

Conversely, the incidence of reported ASD, and related reoperation rates, is biased according to patients' expectation about the outcome and from the surgeons' perception of the technique being used. All together, these nuances introduce noise when evaluating the real and meaningful incidence of ASD in cTDR when compared to ACDF even for single-level disease.

It is clear that the incidence of symptomatic ASD is follow-up-dependent. Only studies with long-term follow-up and/or large patient numbers or meta-analyses can demonstrate statistically significant differences in ASR rates because of the inherently low incidence of adjacent level reoperation (0.66% per year).[9] When the median follow-up from a previous study was extended to 56 months (range: 51–82 months), Nunley and colleagues could demonstrate a clear difference for ASD between cTDR and ACDF.[32] Four meta-analysis by Upadhyaya and colleagues[33] (n = 1098 patients from 3 FDA IDE studies with 2-year follow-up), Wu and colleagues[34] (8 Prospective Randomized Controlled Trials (PRCT), 4-year follow-up), Zhang and colleagues[32] (n = 4516 from 19 PRCT), and Xu and colleagues[35] (11 studies, n = 2632 patients) established a significant risk reduction in the ASR favoring cTDR over ACDF. The rate of ASD was lower in patients who underwent cTDR no matter the follow-up time, and cTDR tended to increase the superiority across time and in 2-level disc disease. It is likely that for more than 2-level cTDR, future research will follow this trend.

Shin reported increasing rates of ASD as more levels were fused (15.38% for 1-level ACDF, 28.57% for 2-level, and 39.47% for 3-level).[36] Laratta and colleagues reported only 6% for ASD revision rate at 24 months for patients who underwent 3- and 4-level fusion.[11] Reinas and colleagues documented (n = 32 patients) that not a single patient had symptomatic ASD leading to reoperation.[24] Regarding cTDR implant-type-related ASD, we still lack long-term follow-up data on third-generation cervical disc prosthesis. It can be hypothesized that implants offering axial compression properties could be more protective against ASD.

Heterotopic Ossification in Multilevel Cervical Total Disc Replacement

The development of HO remains a controversial topic surrounding cervical motion preservation technology. If significant HO occurs, limiting segmental ROM, then cTDR may offer no advantage over fusion. However, as the incidence of HO increases with the duration of follow-up, cTDR may still be beneficial at least during the early years after surgery. On the other hand, most of HO cases do not limit cTDR motion or have negative clinical ramifications.

There is no consensus on the actual incidence of HO after cTDR. This is likely due to the multifactorial nature of HO, reflecting varying patient's pathology, selection criteria, variations in surgical technique, the use of diverse implants, and distinct follow-up periods in different cohorts. According to Tu and colleagues, the incidence of HO maybe more related to the surgical technique than to the concept of motion preservation itself.[37] Exhaustive saline irrigation to eliminate bone dust and removal of posterior longitudinal ligament, abolishing the scaffold for bone growth, may help to reduce HO rates (Pagaimo F, Fernandes P, Xavier J, et al. New methodology to assess in-vivo quality of motion in cervical spine. In submission to Clin Biomech). Inadequate endplate coverage, due to limited disc removal, and postoperative shell kyphosis may also increase the rate of HO (10.3% vs 3.7% grade 4 HO), comparing suboptimal with optimal carpentry.[37] Regarding implant-related HO, Mehren and colleagues[38] revealed that implants with keel anchoring system violating the cortical bone were associated with raised incidence of HO.

The incidence of HO formation after cTDR is also pathology-dependent. It is higher either in patients with spondylosis or calcified discs than in those with a soft-disc herniation[39] or in patients with multilevel disc herniation than in those with a single-level disease after a mean follow-up of 38.3 ± 8.7 months.[40] However, the influence of the number of levels submitted to cTDR on HO is still open to discussion. At 2-year follow-up,

Fig. 3. A 54-year-old female submitted in 2004 to a C5-6 fusion, admitted with neck pain (VAS 5) and L-arm pain (VAS 9, loss of hand dexterity and paresthesia due to adjacent segment disease at C4-5 and C6-7 levels). (A–D) Sagittal and axial T2-weighted cervical MRI showing compression at C4-5 and C6-7 levels; (E, F) Pre-operative dynamic, flexion and extension, lateral cervical radiographs showing previous C5-6 fusion. (G-J) 3-year postoperative dynamic, flexion and extension, lateral cervical radiographs showing 2-level cervical cTDR next to an intermediate level previous fusion. C2-7 and C0-2 angles changed from 15.2° to 18.6° and from 32.2° to 23.3°, respectively, global ROM improved from 20.4° to 30.8°, SVA increased slightly from 14.6mm to 17.9mm, and T1 slope remained roughly unchanged from 36.5° to 36.2° (VAS- visual analogue scale; MRI: magnetic resonance imaging).

Huppert and colleagues found HO to be less prevalent in multilevel than single-level cTDR over 24 months,[22] while Zhao and colleagues found no significant differences between both groups.[41] Gornet and colleagues identified grade 3 or grade 4 HO in 34 of 387 (8.8%) total levels treated with cTDR in 122 patients.[23] In our multilevel cTDR study, when performing a breakdown of HO results between the 2 subgroups, Reinas and colleagues found 8.6% (3/35) of grade I HO in 3- and 4-level patients versus 8.3% (3/39) grade I and 2.7% (1/39) grade II HO in 2-level patients followed up for more than 2 years (range: 24–70 months)[24] (see **Table 1**). Despite the occurrence of HO, the affected functional units not only retained mobility but surprisingly showed a slight increase in ROM at the end of follow-up ($\Delta 3.4 \pm 8.2$ mm, $P = .31$).[24] This may demonstrate that progressive incidence of HO is not incremental with the number of cTDR levels, when using a compressible implant with graded resistance to angular motion. However, the 3- and 4-level cTDR patients enrolled in this cohort were relatively young, with a mean age of 47 years, and predominantly female (10/11).

Durability and Cost-effectiveness of Multilevel Cervical Total Disc Replacement

As cTDR patients tend to be younger than patients compared to ACDF, with an increased life expectancy, questions regarding the durability of cTDR implants are pertinent. In addition, this subgroup of patients may have a more demanding lifestyle imposing increased stress loads, sometimes in extremes of the ROM, on their cervical disc prosthesis. Chen and colleagues[42] in a systematic review and meta-analysis, including 12 randomized Controlled Trials (RCTs) with follow-up from ranging 2 to 7 years, found that cTDR implants, despite their differences in design and materials, are more durable than ACDF. cTDR devices' durability is enhanced by a precise size selection, a proper surgical technique, as well a biomechanical profile that is closer to a normal cervical disc. Wu and colleagues conducted a meta-analysis (based on eight studies with a minimum 4-year follow-up) which demonstrated a significantly higher index level reoperation rate with ACDF (16.8%) than cTDR (7.4%).[34] At the index level, Gornet and colleagues reported 3.6% (5/116) in 3-level cTDR group and no reoperation for the 4-level cTDR group.[23] Laratta and colleagues found a 26% index level reoperation rate for pseudarthrosis for 3- and 4-level ACDF.[11]

If cTDR implants tend to be more expensive than ACDF cages, cTDR is associated with higher durability and less ASR. In the long term (>7 years), cTDR not only optimizes clinical and radiological outcomes compared with ACDF but it is also more cost-effective. The primary driver of the differential in cost-effectiveness is the difference in secondary surgery rates.[43] A study addressing the cost-effectiveness issue found 2-level cTDR to be superior to fusion regarding not only clinical outcomes (greater satisfaction at 2 years of follow-up) but also lower costs over the span of 5 years.[44]

FUTURE DIRECTIONS

Reoperation, at the index or adjacent levels, is a primary inflator of surgery costs. Any comparison of the cost-effectiveness of multilevel cTDR to ACDF requires long-term data to draw valid conclusions. In addition, data on long-term quality of life scores and adverse events should be integrated in cost-effectiveness studies. Ideally, to increase the relevance, these studies should be carried out from real-world data to avoid industry-funding bias. It is also important to dissociate evidence-based clinical safety and efficacy from insurance companies' reimbursement data.

Before instituting widespread cTDR to treat a disease higher than 2-level, it is important to refine cTDR implant design to achieve optimal results. As COR location and load-displacement curves vary in terms of cervical disc location (eg, C3-4 vs C6-7) and patients' age, cTDR design should evolve with custom-made implants to meet different biokinematics requirements. The evolution of the biomechanical properties of the successive generations of cervical disc prosthesis will offer the surgeon the possibility to expand the indications of cTDR to patients suffering from multiple DDD.

CLINICS CARE POINTS

- Although OUS, 3- and 4-level cervical total disc replacement (cTDR) is a compelling option in the surgical armamentarium, it still lacks firm level 1 evidence regarding its effectiveness.

- If the indications of cTDR are to be expanded to 3- and 4-level, it is better to understand the contraindications to reduce complications rates and to meet patients' expectations in the long term.

- Hybrid constructs constitute a valid option for patients with different stages of spondylosis progression. cTDR may be used in less

- spondylotic levels or in those expected to have a higher range of motion.

- Regarding the surgical technique in multi-level cTDR, it is crucial to rely both on direct decompression and proper device insertion to achieve the best biokinematic outcomes that will translate in superior clinical outcomes.

- Devices with a mobile core and compressible property allow a more physiologic center of rotation location and may be advantageous in multilevel cTDR patients.

- The beneficial effect of cTDR on cervical spine alignment may not be inferior to anterior cervical discectomy and fusion (ACDF), as motion preservation allows for proper alignment compensations. This combination is favorable for multilevel cTDR patients.

- The rate of adjacent segment disease and adjacent segment reoperation is lower in multilevel patients who underwent cTDR than ACDF. cTDR superiority increases over time.

- Executing a sound surgical technique, avoiding implants with keels and excluding spondylotic or calcified discs in multilevel disease, may reduce the incidence of heterotopic ossification formation.

ACKNOWLEDGMENTS

The authors would like to thank Ms Sonia Macedo for kindly editing and reviewing this article for English language.

DISCLOSURE

The author has nothing to disclose.

REFERENCES

1. Turel MK, Kerolus MG, Adogwa O, et al. Cervical arthroplasty: what does the labeling say? Neurosurg Focus 2017;42(2):E2.
2. Joaquim AF, Makhni MC, Riew KD. Evidence-based use of arthroplasty in cervical degenerative disc disease. Int Orthop 2019;43(4):767–75.
3. Zhang Y, Liang C, Tao Y, et al. Cervical total disc replacement is superior to anterior cervical decompression and fusion: a meta-analysis of prospective randomized controlled trials. PLoS One 2015;10(3): e0117826.
4. Zou S, Gao J, Xu B, et al. Anterior cervical discectomy and fusion (ACDF) versus cervical disc arthroplasty (CDA) for two contiguous levels cervical disc degenerative disease: a meta-analysis of randomized controlled trials. Eur Spine J 2017; 26(4):985–97.
5. Wang QL, Tu ZM, Hu P, et al. Long-term Results Comparing Cervical Disc Arthroplasty to Anterior Cervical Discectomy and Fusion: A Systematic Review and Meta-Analysis of Randomized Controlled Trials. Orthop Surg 2020;12(1):16–30.
6. Sundseth J, Jacobsen EA, Kolstad F, et al. Heterotopic ossification and clinical outcome in nonconstrained cervical arthroplasty 2 years after surgery: the Norwegian Cervical Arthroplasty Trial (NORCAT). Eur Spine J 2016;25(7):2271–8.
7. Chin-See-Chong TC, Gadjradj PS, Boelen RJ, et al. Current practice of cervical disc arthroplasty: a survey among 383 AOSpine International members. Neurosurg Focus 2017;42(2):E8.
8. Amenta PS, Ghobrial GM, Krespan K, et al. Cervical spondylotic myelopathy in the young adult: a review of the literature and clinical diagnostic criteria in an uncommon demographic. Clin Neurol Neurosurg 2014;120:68–72.
9. Hilibrand AS, Carlson GD, Palumbo MA, et al. Radiculopathy and myelopathy at segments adjacent to the site of a previous anterior cervical arthrodesis. J Bone Joint Surg Am 1999;81(4):519–28.
10. Prasarn ML, Baria D, Milne E, et al. Adjacent-level biomechanics after single versus multilevel cervical spine fusion. J Neurosurg Spine 2012;16(2):172–7.
11. Laratta JL, Reddy HP, Bratcher KR, et al. Outcomes and revision rates following multilevel anterior cervical discectomy and fusion. J Spine Surg 2018;4(3):496–500.
12. Jiang SD, Jiang LS, Dai LY. Anterior cervical discectomy and fusion versus anterior cervical corpectomy and fusion for multilevel cervical spondylosis: a systematic review. Arch Orthop Trauma Surg 2012; 132(2):155–61.
13. Nunley PD, Coric D, Frank KA, et al. Cervical Disc Arthroplasty: Current Evidence and Real-World Application. Neurosurgery 2018;83(6):1087–106.
14. Tetreault L, Wilson JR, Kotter MR, et al. Predicting the minimum clinically important difference in patients undergoing surgery for the treatment of degenerative cervical myelopathy. Neurosurg Focus 2016;40(6):E14.
15. Chang PY, Chang HK, Wu JC, et al. Is cervical disc arthroplasty good for congenital cervical stenosis? J Neurosurg Spine 2017;26(5):577–85.
16. Chang HC, Tu TH, Chang HK, et al. Hybrid Corpectomy and Disc Arthroplasty for Cervical Spondylotic Myelopathy Caused by Ossification of Posterior Longitudinal Ligament and Disc Herniation. World Neurosurg 2016;95:22–30.
17. Roberto RF, McDonald T, Curtiss S, et al. Kinematics of progressive circumferential ligament resection (decompression) in conjunction with cervical disc arthroplasty in a spondylotic spine model. Spine (Phila Pa 1976) 2010;35(18):1676–83.

18. Pimenta L, McAfee PC, Cappuccino A, et al. Superiority of multilevel cervical arthroplasty outcomes versus single-level outcomes: 229 consecutive PCM prostheses. Spine (Phila Pa 1976) 2007;32(12):1337–44.

19. Zhao Y, Zhang Y, Sun Y, et al. Application of Cervical Arthroplasty With Bryan Cervical Disc: 10-Year Follow-up Results in China. Spine (Phila Pa 1976) 2016;41(2):111–5.

20. Chang HK, Huang WC, Tu TH, et al. Radiological and clinical outcomes of 3-level cervical disc arthroplasty. J Neurosurg Spine 2019;32(2):174–81.

21. Joaquim AF, Riew KD. Multilevel cervical arthroplasty: current evidence. A systematic review. Neurosurg Focus 2017;42(2):E4.

22. Huppert J, Beaurain J, Steib JP, et al. Comparison between single- and multi-level patients: clinical and radiological outcomes 2 years after cervical disc replacement. Eur Spine J 2011;20(9):1417–26.

23. Gornet MF, Schranck FW, Sorensen KM, et al. Multi-level Cervical Disc Arthroplasty: Long-Term Outcomes at 3 and 4 Levels. Int J Spine Surg 2020; 14(s2):S41–9.

24. Reinas R, Kitumba D, Pereira L, et al. Multilevel cervical arthroplasty-clinical and radiological outcomes. J Spine Surg 2020;6(1):233–42.

25. Patwardhan AG, Tzermiadianos MN, Tsitsopoulos PP, et al. Primary and coupled motions after cervical total disc replacement using a compressible six-degree-of-freedom prosthesis. Eur Spine J 2012;21(Suppl 5):S618–29.

26. Hung CW, Wu MF, Yu GF, et al. Comparison of sagittal parameters for anterior cervical discectomy and fusion, hybrid surgery, and total disc replacement for three levels of cervical spondylosis. Clin Neurol Neurosurg 2018;168:140–6.

27. Martin S, Ghanayem AJ, Tzermiadianos MN, et al. Kinematics of cervical total disc replacement adjacent to a two-level, straight versus lordotic fusion. Spine (Phila Pa 1976) 2011;36(17):1359–66.

28. Hollyer MA, Gill EC, Ayis S, et al. The safety and efficacy of hybrid surgery for multilevel cervical degenerative disc disease versus anterior cervical discectomy and fusion or cervical disc arthroplasty: a systematic review and meta-analysis. Acta Neurochir (Wien) 2020;162(2):289–303.

29. Lu VM, Mobbs RJ, Phan K. Clinical Outcomes of Treating Cervical Adjacent Segment Disease by Anterior Cervical Discectomy and Fusion Versus Total Disc Replacement: A Systematic Review and Meta-Analysis. Glob Spine J 2019;9(5):559–67.

30. Sekhon LH, Sears W, Duggal N. Cervical arthroplasty after previous surgery: results of treating 24 discs in 15 patients. J Neurosurg Spine 2005;3(5):335–41.

31. Cunningham BW, Hu N, Zorn CM, et al. Biomechanical comparison of single- and two-level cervical arthroplasty versus arthrodesis: effect on adjacent-level spinal kinematics. Spine J 2010;10(4):341–9.

32. Nunley PD, Jawahar A, Cavanaugh DA, et al. Symptomatic adjacent segment disease after cervical total disc replacement: re-examining the clinical and radiological evidence with established criteria. Spine J 2013;13(1):5–12.

33. Upadhyaya CD, Wu JC, Trost G, et al. Analysis of the three United States Food and Drug Administration investigational device exemption cervical arthroplasty trials. J Neurosurg Spine 2012;16(3): 216–28.

34. Wu TK, Liu H, Wang BY, et al. Minimum four-year subsequent surgery rates of cervical disc replacement versus fusion: A meta-analysis of prospective randomized clinical trials. Orthop Traumatol Surg Res 2017;103(1):45–51.

35. Xu S, Liang Y, Zhu Z, et al. Adjacent segment degeneration or disease after cervical total disc replacement: a meta-analysis of randomized controlled trials. J Orthop Surg Res 2018;13(1):244.

36. Shin JJ. Comparison of Adjacent Segment Degeneration, Cervical Alignment, and Clinical Outcomes After One- and Multilevel Anterior Cervical Discectomy and Fusion. Neurospine 2019;16(3):589–600.

37. Tu TH, Wu JC, Huang WC, et al. The effects of carpentry on heterotopic ossification and mobility in cervical arthroplasty: determination by computed tomography with a minimum 2-year follow-up: Clinical article. J Neurosurg Spine 2012;16(6):601–9.

38. Mehren C, Wuertz-Kozak K, Sauer D, et al. Implant Design and the Anchoring Mechanism Influence the Incidence of Heterotopic Ossification in Cervical Total Disc Replacement at 2-year Follow-up. Spine (Phila Pa 1976) 2019;44(21):1471–80.

39. Wu JC, Huang WC, Tu TH, et al. Differences between soft-disc herniation and spondylosis in cervical arthroplasty: CT-documented heterotopic ossification with minimum 2 years of follow-up. J Neurosurg Spine 2012;16(2):163–71.

40. Wu JC, Huang WC, Tsai HW, et al. Differences between 1- and 2-level cervical arthroplasty: more heterotopic ossification in 2-level disc replacement: Clinical article. J Neurosurg Spine 2012;16(6): 594–600.

41. Zhao H, Cheng L, Hou Y, et al. Multi-level cervical disc arthroplasty (CDA) versus single-level CDA for the treatment of cervical disc diseases: a meta-analysis. Eur Spine J 2015;24(1):101–12.

42. Chen C, Zhang X, Ma X. Durability of cervical disc arthroplasties and its influence factors: A systematic review and a network meta-analysis. Medicine (Baltimore) 2017;96(6):e5947.

43. Radcliff K, Guyer RD. Economics of Cervical Disc Replacement. Int J Spine Surg 2020;14(s2):S67–72.

44. Health Quality Ontario. Cervical Artificial Disc Replacement Versus Fusion for Cervical Degenerative Disc Disease: A Health Technology Assessment. Ont Health Technol Assess Ser 2019;19(3):1–223.

Cervical Total Disc Replacement: Novel Devices

Richard D. Guyer, MD[a],*, Joseph L. Albano, DO[b], Donna D. Ohnmeiss, PhD[c]

KEYWORDS

- Cervical disc arthroplasty • Cervical disc replacement • Novel devices • Cervical spine
- Radiculopathy • Myelopathy • Spine surgery

KEY POINTS

- Cervical disc arthroplasty demonstrates superior pain and disability results to anterior cervical discectomy and fusion.
- Cervical disc arthroplasty demonstrates a 3- to 4-fold decrease in revision surgery.
- Third-generation cervical disc arthroplasty allow 6° of freedom from viscoelastic core.
- Some newer iterations of cervical disc arthroplasty use MRI-compatible materials for postoperative imaging.
- Few novel cervical disc arthroplasty implants are available for use in the United States.

INTRODUCTION

Over the course of the last several decades, cervical disc arthroplasty (CDA) has emerged as a surgical alternative for cervical myelopathy and radiculopathy. Compared with anterior cervical discectomy and fusion (ACDF), CDA has been shown to be superior in clinical outcomes for neck pain and disability at two and 4 years and more closely resemble native motion of the cervical spine.[1–6] CDA has also been shown to have lower reoperation and readmission rates over a 30-day period as well as over 5 years.[7,8] A major reason for this is the ability to maintain or even restore motion to a diseased cervical spine segment to more closely resemble the native spine, without significantly affecting the adjacent levels.[3,5,9–11]

One of the principle concerns with regard to any spinal fusion procedure is the likelihood of affecting the adjacent segments. It has been demonstrated by Jackson and colleagues[8] that as far out as 60 months from index procedure, CDA results in up to a four-fold decrease in adjacent level revision surgery, most likely due to preservation of motion. While it is known that fusion results in increased motion at adjacent levels, motion, as well as intradiscal pressure, tends to be preserved in CDA.[12–14] Flexion tends to be maintained to near-normal limits, whereas lateral bending has a 40%-60% decrease in motion compared with a native segment with implantation of a CDA device.[13–15] As a result of this improved, but nonphysiologic, motion, it is postulated that increased loading of the facet joints at the implanted levels, owing to greater flexibility, but an unloading at the level above.[16,17] Notwithstanding, some of these implants, such as the ProDisc-C (Centinel Spine, West Chester, PA), transmit load through their mobile core, leading to a decrease in facet and uncovertebral joint load transmission.

BIOMECHANICAL CONSIDERATIONS

The biomechanics of spine arthroplasty have changed throughout the development of various technologies. Compared to the lumbar disc, a

a Center for Disc Replacement at Texas Back Institute, 6020 W. Parker Rd. #200, Plano, TX 75093, USA; b Texas Back Institute, 6020 W. Parker Rd. #200, Plano, TX 75093, USA; c Texas Back Institute Research Foundation, 6020 W. Parker Rd. #200, Plano, TX 75093, USA
* Corresponding author.
E-mail address: rguyer@texasback.com

Neurosurg Clin N Am 32 (2021) 449–460
https://doi.org/10.1016/j.nec.2021.05.004

native cervical disc carries 1/9 the load of its lumbar counterpart, and therefore, the biomechanical considerations are unique to this region.[18] Originally arthroplasty technology was broadly classified into constrained and semi-constrained prosthesis, owing to the extent of motion allowed by a particular implant.[19,20] This classification can be further described by number of components and degrees of freedom, which include flexion/extension, lateral sidebending, axial rotation, translation in the anterior-posterior and lateral directions, and compression.[21]

The original designs for CDA were modeled after large joint arthroplasty and therefore fail to fully capture the dynamic motion in the cervical spine.[22] The Prestige was the first cervical disc in the United States released in 2007 which consisted of a metal-on-metal, noncongruent, articulating ball and socket joint, which allowed some translation during flexion and extension. When Mobi-C was released, it was the first with a mobile core that allowed translation. It translates in the A-P and lateral directions, allowing for a total of 5° of freedom. The only motion that is not possible with the Mobi-C is compression through the device, due to its solid core.

These original iterations alter the mechanics of the involved spine segment by bringing the center of rotation in flexion/extension and lateral side bending more caudal.[21] As these motions are coupled, failure of one of the articulations will impede motion in other planes. For example, with regard to the Mobi-C, the mobile core translates anterior, and if it sticks or ceases to move, flexion and extension will be limited, putting more stress on the facet joints or on the bone-implant interface.[21] In addition, the center of rotation in lateral bending with these mobile core devices is altered, leading to facet abutment and the potential for further pain and degeneration.[21] Contrarily, as degrees of freedom are increased, stability tends to decrease, which would impart greater stress on the surrounding soft-tissue structures causing facet and uncovertebral degeneration.[22]

THIRD-GENERATION CERVICAL DISC ARTHROPLASTY

The third generation of disc arthroplasty technology involve implants that allow for all 6° of freedom, including compression. The M6-C (Orthofix Medical Inc.; Lewisville, TX), Baguera-C (Spine Art Inc; Geneva, Switzerland), Rhine (Stryker, Leesburg, VA) and CP-ESP (Spinal Innovations, Hemisbrunn, France) all have so-called nonarticulating components, which allow motion

in all planes while offering unique internal resistance mechanisms to confer stability.[21]

Another hurdle for arthroplasty technology to overcome with its newer iterations is the compatibility with imaging such as CT and MRI. Implants such as the Simplify-C and Baguera-C are composed of imaging compatible materials such as polyetheretherketone (PEEK), polyethylene, and diamond-like-carbon (DLC)-coated titanium. The M-6 is titanium, and the Prestige LP is a composite of titanium and ceramic which also have reasonable imaging but still do produce some artifact on CT and MRI.

M6-C

The M6-C (**Fig. 1**), initially implanted in 2005, is one of the most widely used nonarticulating, compressible core implants in the market today with over 50,000 cervical and lumbar discs implanted. It was approved for use by the Federal Drug Administration (FDA) in 2019 in the United States.

The M6-C has a mobile bumper design, meaning the endplates are not firmly bonded to its polycarbonate urethane (PCU) core. The core, which is meant to replicate the nucleus, is surrounded by a woven-fiber ultra-high-molecular-weight polyethylene (UHWMPE) to serve as a substitute for the annulus, which is laser-welded to the titanium endplates.[22] The core and UHMWPE fibers are all surrounded by a PCU sheath to prevent extrusion of debris into the surrounding environment and to prevent ingrowth of tissue into the implant. The endplates are sprayed with a titanium plasma spray to promote bony ingrowth.

Owing to its compressible core, 6° of freedom are possible with the M6-C implant; however, it is not completely unconstrained because of its annular fibers. These UHMWPE fibers provide a bending resistance to the implant, which may be important in restoring bending stiffness in a hypermobile disc.[21] Amadji and colleagues describes the M6-C as demonstrating equivalent quality of motion, compared with healthy discs, and notes the artificial fiber annulus and nucleus as critical in this function.[23] The kinematic signature, in other words, the applied moment versus the segmental angular motion, of the M6-C has been shown to be similar to a native cervical disc.[21] This is due to the built-in bending stiffness of the prosthesis with the coupled surrounding soft-tissue tensioning. Owing to its inherent resistance to motion, resection of the PLL has not been shown to affect motion after implantation of the M6-C.[21]

Patwardhan and colleagues[24] looked at the primary and coupled motion in cadaveric specimens

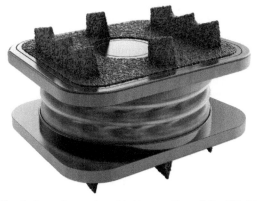
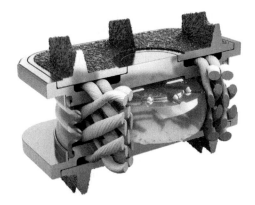

Fig. 1. Posterior and sagittal transection of the M6-C implant showing the PCU core surrounded by a woven-fiber ultra-high-molecular-weight-polyethylene (UHWMPE). The core and UHMWPE fibers are all surrounded by a PCU sheath. (Image provided courtesy of Orthofix Medical Inc, Lewisville, TX with permission.)

implanted with the M6. They found that while flexion and extension range of motion were maintained, lateral bending and axial rotation of implanted segments decreased, which has been described with other implants as well.[24] Despite its similarity in motion of a native disc, the axis of rotation of the compressible core prostheses, such as the M6-C, is located caudal and cranial in flexion/extension and lateral bending, respectively.[21] Therefore, despite its ability to accommodate near-physiologic motion, the lack of lateral bending of approximately 40° noted may come from an inability of the prostheses to accommodate the additional translation required for these altered axes of rotation.[21] Compared with the Mobi-C prosthesis, Pham and colleagues[11] described a decrease in overall extension but maintained flexion, yet both were equal at the C6/7 level. Notwithstanding, no differences were found in either clinical or radiographic outcomes with a mean follow-up duration of 29 months.[25]

Implantation of the M6-C has been shown in several studies to improve pain, function, and quality of life, as well as preserve normal range of motion of the segment.[3,26–28] It has emerged as a surgical option for radiculopathy and myelopathy with a great deal of success evidenced by its large number of implanted devices. There have also been several documented complications which warrant further investigation. One case report of the PCU core herniating posteriorly, with rupture of the posterior structures 8 years after implantation causing signs of myelopathy, was described in 2014. The implant was removed with the segment fused with gradual resolution of symptoms.[29] Another case described rupture of the component with thread extrusion and a granulomatous reaction surrounding the ruptured fragments.[30]

In addition, periprosthetic osteolysis and late-onset infections are beginning to emerge as potential long-term complications of this device, requiring revision to a fusion.[31,32] This is an area requiring further investigation and may be a result of the UHMWPE annulus or the core and sheath interaction with the local microenvironment. In fact, as of February 6, 2020, the Australian Government issued a safety warning regarding the increased incidence of osteolysis causing failure noted after implantation of M6-C implants.

CP-ESP

The CP-ESP prosthesis (**Fig. 2**) is another example of a nonarticulating, one-component CDA allowing for all 6° of freedom. While the lumbar counterpart was approved for use in Europe in 2005, the CP-ESP obtained Conformitè Europëenne (CE) approval in 2012.[4] It consists of a polyurethane carbonate core, designed to mimic the natural motion of a native cervical disc and also impart

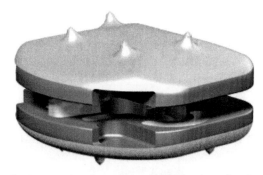

Fig. 2. Anterior view of the CP-ESP implant showing the polyurethane carbonate core between the hydroxyapatite-coated endplates. (Image provided courtesy of Spine Innovations, Hemisbrunn, France with permission.)

resistance to motion.[4,22] The core is well fixed to the endplates via adhesion molding, which is a potential site for shear forces and debonding.[22] As a means of additional supplementation, there are male and female pegs within the implant to control compression, translation, and shear.[4] The endplates have spikes to provide primary fixation, as well as a hydroxyapatite coating to improve on growth.[4] The design was based on a model that focused on stiffness rather than mobility to mimic natural disc movement, to avoid overloading the facet joints.[4] As a result, the biomechanics of this implant approach that of a normal human disc.[4] In vitro analysis demonstrates flexion/extension of 14° of motion and 12°and 8° of lateral bending and axial rotation, respectively, which is similar to that of the native spine.[4,21] In terms of fatigue, the CP-ESP disc resulted in decreased loss of disc height compared with other implants, without significant variation in endplate alignment.[4] The PCU was assessed for wear relating to aging, which was also found to be insignificant.

Lazennec and colleagues evaluated 62 patients in their preliminary study with 74% and 26% at single and two levels, respectively.[4] At one and 2 years, there were no device-related complications including malalignment, instability, or heterotopic ossification.[4] Range of motion of the instrumented and adjacent levels demonstrated maintenance of acceptable range of motion up to 2 years.[4] All patients were improved from their preoperative condition. They conceded that longer term follow-up would be necessary.

Rhine

The Rhine arthroplasty device (**Fig. 3**) demonstrates another 6° of freedom, nonarticulating implant. It was approved for use in Europe in 2016 and had 300 devices implanted by the end of 2017. The core, composed of a polyurethane

like the CP-ESP, is intended to mimic the mechanics of stiffness and strength of a healthy cervical disc.[14] Its titanium endplates are plasma sprayed to increase integration with the bony endplates.[14] In a cadaveric model, the Rhine CDA demonstrated physiologic flexion and extension motion with optimal position.[14,22] Consistent with the literature, there was a decrease in lateral bending and axial rotation to 42% and 57% of normal.[14] Slight anterior or lateral placement demonstrated motion similar to optimal placement, indicating a potential for suboptimal placement and satisfactory results.[14]

Freedom

The Freedom CDA implant (**Fig. 4**) is a one-component, nonarticulating arthroplasty device with 6° of freedom. It received the CE mark in 2012 for use in the European Union. It has a viscoelastic PCU core bonded to the titanium endplates, which are porous bead-coated.[33] It is a more developed iteration of Axiomed's lumbar disc arthroplasty, Acroflex, which had a polyolefin rubber core that demonstrated in vivo tears in 36% of patients.[22] The core bonds to the endplates by a variety of mechanisms including chemical bonding, titanium beads that interlock with the core, and a raised ridge and wedged endplates to decrease shear.[22]

There is one study with 2-year clinical data in one- and two-level patients. The authors conclude decreases in visual analog scale (VAS) and Neck Disability Index (NDI) scores immediately postoperatively to 2 years. There were no patients with worsening symptoms. Patient satisfaction was

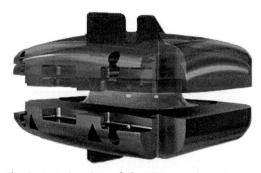

Fig. 3. Anterior view of the Rhine implant showing the plasma-sprayed titanium end and polyurethane core. (Image provided courtesy of Stryker Spine, Leesburg, Virginia with permission.)

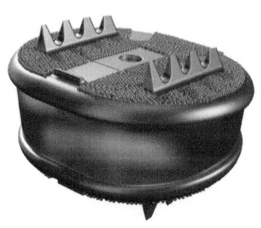

Fig. 4. Anterior view of the Freedom implant demonstrating the porous bead-coated titanium endplates and polyolefin rubber core bonded to the endplates. (Image provided courtesy of Axiomed, Malden, MA with permission.)

increased at the 2-year postoperative visits in 83% of patients.[34] The authors conclude that these results are similar to other studies looking at articulating and viscoelastic CDAs.[34] However, as Jacobs and colleagues[22] mention, the study only evaluates patient-reported outcomes and does not evaluate device-related complications. Axiomed's analysis of biocompatibility also demonstrates that if any particulate is generated from this device, it does not cause an inflammatory response, and that long-term simulated in vivo exposure does not change the material properties of the device.[35]

MRI COMPATIBLE DEVICES
Baguera-C

The Baguera-C CDA (**Fig. 5**) is unique in that it is a three-component device that allows for 6° of freedom. It has been approved for use since 2007, in Europe, and is anticipating to initiate their one- and two-level FDA Investigation Device Exemption (IDE) trials in 2021. Baguera-C had successfully implanted over 15,000 devices. The endplates of the Baguera-C are made of titanium and coated with a diamond-like (Diamolith) interior and porous-coated exterior.[36] The DLC interior serves to decrease wear while also having low friction and is also more MRI compatible than other titanium implants.[37] The nucleus is a UHMWPE insert, which rests in the inferior endplate and articulates with the superior endplate. This device allows compression in the form of elastic deformation of the inferior endplate and the UHWMPE core in

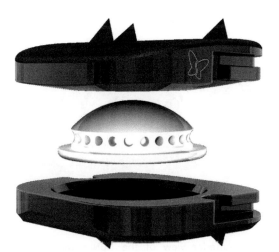

Fig. 5. Posterior view of the Baguera C showing the white mobile and compressible core inside the titanium-coated diamond-like endplates. (Image provided courtesy of Spineart USA Inc, Laguna Hills, CA with permission.)

the amount of 0.15 mm to absorb shock and vibrations, compared to 0.5 mm of compression with the M6-C device.[36,38] The controlled motion of the nucleus prevents excessive constraint on the facets.[38]

Compared with the ProDisc-C Nova and Discocerv CDA implants, the Baguera-C demonstrated wider distribution of contact area and lower contact pressure. There was also no lift-off phenomenon noted with the Baguera-C compared with those other two devices.[39] However, only the flexion moment mimicked a healthy cervical disc in terms of center of rotation.[39] Notwithstanding, the authors of this biomechanical analysis considered the Baguera-C biomechanically superior to the ProDisc-C Nova and Discocerv implants.[39] Several studies have demonstrated improvement in patient-reported VAS and NDI scores at 2 years with no device-related complications.[38,40] It was also found that patients younger than 50 years, without prior spine or other cervical conditions surgery, and no preoperative functional disabilities demonstrated superior results.[36]

Heo and colleagues investigated bone loss of the operative level vertebral bodies.[41] They found that 29 out of 48 patients observed in their analysis who were treated with the Baguera-C implant developed some degree of bone loss associated with postoperative neck pain; however, it did not affect mid- to long-term clinical outcomes and may have resulted in the motion preservation effect of the operative segment.[41] Kieser and colleagues also looked that this phenomenon and found that, when looking at multiple implants over a 5-year follow-up, most bone loss was mild in nature.[42] They conclude that age, sex, postoperative alignment, range of motion, and midflexion point do not relate to this phenomenon, but the number of levels operated on does contribute to this. They found no long-term effect on the mechanical function of the disc.[42]

Simplify Cervical Artificial Disc

While it is not a device which allows 6° of freedom, the Simplify CDA (**Fig. 6**) demonstrates an attempt to improve some of the drawbacks of other, earlier products. It offers smaller implants to avoid overstuffing, allowing for devices with a height as low as 4 mm, which may be ideal in particularly collapsed levels. Additionally offered are 5° lordotic options for some of its larger implants, to help potentially correct or match the patients natural lordosis. The Simplify disc was approved for use in Europe in 2015, and as of September, 2020, it was approved for use by the FDA for single-level disease in the United States. They

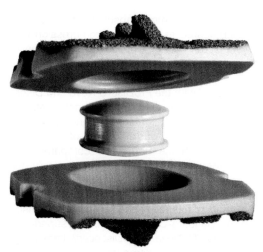

Fig. 6. Posterior view of the Simplify Cervical Disc Arthroplasty with titanium-sprayed PEEK endplates with concavities for the zirconia toughened alumina ceramic mobile core. (Image provided courtesy of Simplify Medical, Sunnyvale, CA with permission.)

have also completed their two-level IDE study and have submitted for premarket approval, which will likely be granted in the coming months. One obstacle in particular it seeks to overcome is artifact on postoperative imagine. The product is made from MRI-compatible materials which reduce scatter to enhance imaging after surgery. While other products on the market contain metals such as titanium and cobalt-chrome preventing clear postoperative assessment with MRI at the surgical site and adjacent levels, the aim of these materials is to allow continued diagnosis and appropriate treatment after the index procedure.[43,44]

The endplates are made of PEEK coated with a titanium plasma spray to permit ongrowth, along with superior spikes and an inferior keel to allow for initial fixation in the endplates. The mobile core is comprised of zirconia toughened alumina ceramic and is biconvex in shape with a cylindrical center to allow articulation with the concave internal surfaces of the superior and inferior endplates. There is also a retention ring around the endplate articulations to prevent expulsion of the core. This design allows for translation in both the AP and lateral planes as well as flexion/extension, lateral bending, and axial rotation. The articulation of the ceramic mobile core on the PEEK endplates has been shown to be a reasonable alternative to polyethylene on cobalt chrome and metal-on-metal bearings currently used.[45] Additionally demonstrated were acceptable wear rates with respect to size and morphology of particulate compared with other similar orthopedic couples.[45]

NuNec

The NuNec cervical disc replacement by Surgalign (**Fig. 7**) was initially approved in Europe in 2008 and, as of October of 2012, had 2000 devices implanted. It is a two-component device with endplates made of PEEK-coated hydroxyapatite for long-term osseous integration.[46] The two components articulate in a ball-in-socket conformation. Different than many other CDAs, the NuNec device has a convex superior articulation and a concave component inferiorly. This has implications in terms of the segmental center of rotation compared with other devices with a fixed core and should theoretically raise the center of rotation. The PEEK endplates achieve immediate fixation with a titanium cam which has blades that can carve into the vertebral endplate. There are two of these on the inferior component, and one superiorly. The cams have an aspect without blades so it can be inserted into a milled hole and then rotated similar to a screw to integrate into the vertebral endplate. Because the core is fixed to the superior endplate, there is no translation allotted, and therefore only has 3° of freedom (flexion/extension, lateral bending, and rotation). Wear analysis of this PEEK-on-PEEK articulation demonstrated 1.0-mg-per million cycles.[46] Another bench study found that the NuNec implant uses boundary lubrication regime with the generation of wear debris.[47] There was a maximum contact stress of 32.1 MPal, which is well under the PEEK fatigue strength of 400G.[47]

Japanese Orthopaedic Association pain scores and VAS scores were shown to improve over a 6-month period, with an increase in segmental

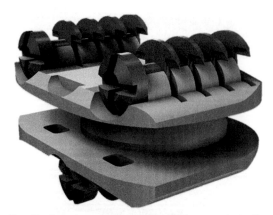

Fig. 7. Anterior view of the NuNec cervical disc replacement with hydroxyapatite-coated PEEK endplates. In pink are the titanium cam blades to achieve immediate fixation in the endplates. (Image provided courtesy of Surgalign Spine Technologies, Deerfield, IL with permission.)

ROM and disc height.[48] The 2-year clinical data for NuNec showed comparable results to other disc arthroplasties. While the range of motion was decreased with this implant, there were higher rates of heterotopic ossification, and there was a very low reoperation rate.[49]

NEXT TO BEGIN IDE TRIAL
Synergy

The Synergy Disc Replacement is a solid core device that allows 4° of freedom with safety stops in all planes to offer some constraint (**Fig. 8**). Compared to the Mobi-C, it does not allow for lateral translation. Its endplates are made of titanium with a plasma spray and three rows of a hybrid of teeth and keels for provisional fixation. The core is UHMWPE and is offered in a zero- or six-degree lordotic option, which they tout provides the ability to preserve or correct sagittal alignment. The company also states that this is the first disc to offer physiologic center of rotation. As of January 29, 2021, they enrolled their first patient in their IDE study.

In a study by Lazaro and colleagues, the Synergy Disc increased the anterior and posterior disc heights and demonstrated the least variability in the shell angle, or the angle between the superior and inferior endplates, while maintaining adequate range of motion.[50] Clearly, a differentiating factor in this competitive space, the lordotic core, has also been shown to maintain an endplate angle of 6° ± 2.7° two years postoperatively, comparable to corrections found with traditional ACDF.[51,52] While the Simplify Cervical Disc (described elsewhere in the article) is the first to market to introduce lordotic endplate options for some of its sizes, analogous to some of its lumbar

counterparts, the Synergy Disc Replacement is the first to introduce a lordotic mobile core, which perhaps explains the advertised physiologic center of rotation in all planes. It will, however, only be offered in a 5-mm and 6-mm height.

Triadyme-C

The Triadyme-C (**Fig. 9**) by Dymicron is the next CDA set to begin its IDE enrollment. It was first implanted abroad in 2015. This device is unique in its articulations and the materials it is made of. It is a two-component, trilobed design, which allows for 5° of freedom, including anterior-posterior and lateral translation. It does not allow for compression. The endplates are titanium with two keels on each endplate for immediate fixation, while a porous titanium plasma spray coating allows for secondary fixation. The inner articulations of each endplate are made of polycrystalline diamond (PCD), which is a diamond-like material that yields lower wear rates and superior structural integrity than other substances used in CDAs.[53] The layers are fully fused and chemically bonded to each other.

The articulations are tri-lobed, with three convex articulations on the cephalad component and three concave articulations on the caudal component. Because the radii of the lobes are smaller than the corresponding pockets in each of the three articulations, there are greater contact stresses imparted by physiologic movement.[21,53] Furthermore, while these articulations may cause high volumes of wear debris in other arthroplasties using UHMWPE or ceramics, the PCD is resistant to wear under such loads.[53] In a biomechanics study by Havey and colleagues,[53] the Triadyme-C restored flexion/extension motion to that of intact levels with only moderate segmental

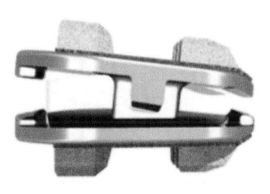 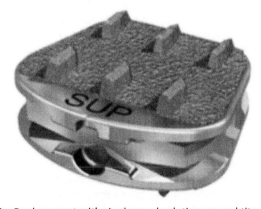

Fig. 8. Lateral and anterosuperior views of the Synergy Disc Replacement with six-degree lordotic core and titanium endplates with plasma spray coating. (Image provided courtesy of Synergy Spine Solutions Louisville, CO with permission.)

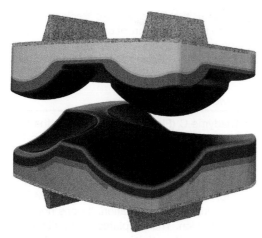

Fig. 9. Oblique view of the Triadyme-C with titanium endplates with porous titanium plasma spray coating, and polycrystalline diamond (PCD), trilobed articulations. (Image provided courtesy of Dymicron, Orem, UT with permission.)

stiffness. Because the implant is so new to the market, there are no available clinical data.

NO ENDPLATE
Cadisc-C

The Cadisc-C is another example of a nonarticulating, one-component prosthesis made of polycarbonate-polyurethane. Although this disc has been discontinued because of issues in particular with the lumbar design, it is important to note the advances in technology present with this device. The surface is coated with calcium phosphate to enhance osteointegration. While the Cadisc-C was granted the CE mark in 2011, it was pulled in 2014 because of a high rate of revision (nearly 50%) in its lumbar counterpart. The company, Ranier Technology, was dissolved in 2018 after further reports of migration and disintegration of the disc. As it has no metal endplates, it is conducive to postoperative imaging with MRI reducing artifact and enhancing postoperative evaluation. It has a graduated modulus with a lower modulus nucleus and higher modules annular region to mimic the native disc and to prevent a sharp interface between materials of different properties.[54,55] There are no bonding regions, and therefore a low risk of producing debris.[22]

While there have been no published studies regarding the Cadisc-C, there have been two studies looking at the biomechanical behavior of the lumbar version, Cadisc-L. Mahomed and colleagues evaluated twelve Cadisc-L samples and found that flexural stiffness increased linearly

with compressive load but decreased with flexural rate, similar to the native lumbar spine.[55] Axial stiffness was also found to decrease by approximately 50% with the Cadisc-L in a laboratory simulation, whereas flexion stiffness was not significantly altered.[54] There is one case report indicating a failure wherein a disc herniation of the Cadisc-L itself led to compression of the posterior neural elements.[56] They were initially treated with microscopic sequestrectomy of the arthroplasty material but presented less than a month later with recurrent symptoms and underwent excision of the arthroplasty and a front-back fusion construct with a cage with resolution of symptoms.[56]

FUTURE DIRECTIONS
Granvia-C

The Granvia-C (**Fig. 10**) implant is produced by Medicrea, who were recently acquired by Medtronic in July of 2020, obtained the CE mark in 2010. The endplates are zirconia ceramic and have chevron ridges to allow for bony fixation, and the roughened surface allows for osteointegration. The core is made of ceramic and PEEK serving as a shock absorber. The superior endplate is concave allowing for the spherical superior aspect of the core to rotate axially as well as engage in flexion/extension and lateral bending. The inferior endplate has a cylindrical trough to allow for lateral bending only. While the compression of this device does not allow as much motion as other one prosthesis products, it does allow for shock absorption. Owing to its ceramic and PEEK components, it is ideal for postoperative MRI scans. There was one abstract presented on the Granvia-C, which evaluated 18 patients implanted with the device in one or two levels. They reported

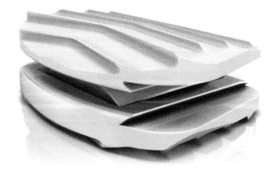

Fig. 10. Posterior view of the Granvia-C implant with zirconia ceramic endplates with chevron ridges. The core is made of ceramic and PEEK and serves as a shock absorber. (Image provided courtesy of Medtronic, Minneapolis, MN with permission.)

improvement in VAS and NDI over their 6-month follow-up, without any device-related complications.[57] They also reported no MRI artifact on the 5 patients that had postoperative MRI scans. As of 2015, the Granvia-C began enrollment in a multicenter European pilot study.

Neophytos

The Neophytos CDA, which is produced in Cyprus, Greece, is relatively new and is another iteration of the one component device, allowing 6° of freedom. It has titanium endplates with spikes superiorly and inferiorly allowing initial fixation and are coated with hydroxyapatite to allow bone in growth. The core is bonded to the endplates and is composed of silicone. There are no publications regarding this implant yet, as it is so new, but the company boasts that it has been tested in the laboratory to endure at least 5,000,000 cycles.

D-Flex

The D-Flex (**Fig. 11**) by Norm Medical is another example of a compressible disc. There are two iterations of this implant, one with titanium endplates (D-Flex-Titanium), and one with PEEK Carbon endplates (D-Flex-Carbon) with the added benefit of MRI compatibility. The core in both of these implants is made of silicon to allow for compressibility. There are not yet any published data on these devices.

MOVE-C

The MOVE-C (**Fig. 12**) CDA from NGMedical is another example of a new implant with 6° of

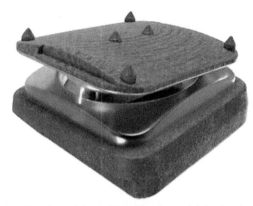

Fig. 12. View of the MOVE-C implant with its titanium alloy cranial and caudal endplates. The caudal endplate has an injection molded polycarbonate-urethane (PCU) core allowing articulation with the cranial endplate. (Image provided courtesy of NG Medical, Nonnweiler Germany with permission.)

freedom. The device received its CE approval in December of 2019 and was first implanted in January of 2020. The cranial and caudal endplates are made of a titanium alloy with spokes at the center and corners for initial endplate adherence, with the caudal endplate having an injection molded PCU allowing articulation with the cranial endplate.[58] With the PCU bearing fixed to the caudal implant, the concave articulation of the cranial implant together serves as a compressible ball and socket joint.[58] The MOVE-C was subject to many biomechanical and wear tests demonstrating acceptable wear (1.38–1.54 mg per million cycles).[58] In addition, the creep and relaxation curve demonstrated a physiologic J-shaped curve as in the human disc, demonstrating the implants' ability to recover following creep.[58]

Secure C3

The Secure-C implant from Globus Medical has been available for use in the United States since 2012 and is a commonly used product. The newest iteration from this product line is the Secure C3, a device which touts both MRI compatibility and 6° of freedom. The endplates are made of coated PEEK. The central keel has 3 spikes to ensure implant stability. The articulation is PEEK on PEEK to generate low-volume wear compared with metal-on-metal or metal-on-polyethylene, and the core is made of PCU to allow compressibility. The Secure-3C is not yet approved for use in the United States.

SUMMARY

The evolution of CDA devices has undergone multiple iterations throughout its decades-long

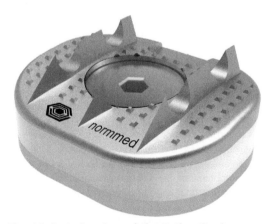

Fig. 11. Posterior view of the D-Flex titanium seen here with titanium endplates and silicone core for compressibility. Not pictured is the D-Flex Carbon implant with carbon fiber endplates for enhanced imaging quality. (Image provided courtesy of Norm Medical Yenimahalle, Turkey with permission.)

history. Since the first of the CDAs, we have learned a great deal about the biomechanics of native and artificial discs that have allowed us to improve on older designs. One thing, however, that has been consistent throughout the literature is the improvement with regard to patient reports outcomes and need for future surgery compared to the gold standard ACDF.[1–8] As newer designs continue to emerge, it will be important to rigorously evaluate these devices with regard to biomechanical and clinical outcomes, learning from the lessons that have been borne out in the literature in the cervical disc's history. It is certainly a fast-evolving aspect of spine surgery, and one in which we can build future technologies with superb patient outcomes in mind. With a variety of new implants in the development pipeline, we will need to make sure they are held to the rigorous standards of their predecessors.

What has not been addressed to date is determining the proper fit of the implant and uniformity. The human disc endplates vary from person to person in height, shape, and concavity. Despite the availability of various heights from the different manufacturers, some of the endplates are flat, some convex, some round, and others trapezoidal. So, a 5-mm height in one disc may not equal a 5 mm in another. Asian patients in general require smaller disc heights than most discs provide.[59] The market is however moving toward smaller and more customizable implants, as the new Simplify Cervical Artificial Disc is the only implant to offer a 4-mm option. In addition, in a study evaluating the fit of multiple cervical disc arthroplasties by Thaler, most implants were undersized relative to the actual dimensions of the endplates, especially in the anterior-posterior direction. This has the potential to allow for subsidence due to inadequate fit and lack of contact with the ring apophysis.[60] Ideally, in the future, we will be able to have patient-specific implants. All these variables can then be accounted for. Unlike fusion, cervical arthroplasties need to adjust to the patient-specific anatomy and biomechanics.

CLINICS CARE POINTS

- Native cervical motion is inherently coupled owing to the viscoelastic nature of the cervical disc.
- Irrespective of having an endplate, all cervical disc arthroplasty (CDA) devices demonstrate a decrease in lateral bending of 40%-60%.

- The M6-C demonstrates a similar kinematic signature to a native cervical disc in vitro.
- M6-C is the only viscoelastic CDA approved for use in the United States.
- There is increasing evidence of osteolysis with the M6-C implant, as evidenced by the warning from the Australian Government.
- The Simplify Cervical Artificial Disc is the first MRI compatible implant, with PEEK component, approved for use in the United States as of September, 2020, and is available in a 4-mm height.
- The Baguera-C began its Federal Drug Administration IDE study as of August 2020 and is also made of MRI-compatible components.
- The CP-ESP and Freedom CDAs have shown favorable patient-related results in European studies.

DISCLOSURE

Some of the authors of this article have commercial or financial disclosures. Please see the attached disclosure forms. There was no funding received for the publication of this article.

REFERENCES

1. Sasso RC, Anderson PA, Riew KD, et al. Results of cervical arthroplasty compared with anterior discectomy and fusion: four-year clinical outcomes in a prospective, randomized controlled trial. J Bone Joint Surg Am 2011;93:1684–92.
2. Sasso RC, Smucker JD, Hacker RJ, et al. Artificial disc versus fusion: a prospective, randomized study with 2-year follow-up on 99 patients. Spine 2007;32: 2933–40.
3. Reyes-Sanchez A, Miramontes V, Olivarez LMR, et al. Initial clinical experience with a next-generation artificial disc for the treatment of symptomatic degenerative cervical radiculopathy. SAS J 2010;4:9–15.
4. Lazennec JY, Aaron A, Ricart O, et al. The innovative viscoelastic CP ESP cervical disk prosthesis with six degrees of freedom: biomechanical concepts, development program and preliminary clinical experience. Eur J Orthop Surg Traumatol 2016;26:9–19.
5. Gandhi AA, Grosland NM, Kallemeyn NA, et al. Biomechanical analysis of the cervical spine following disc degeneration, disc fusion, and disc replacement: A finite element study. Int J Spine Surg 2019;13:491–500.
6. Ohnmeiss D, Guyer R, Samocha Y, et al. Cervical total disc replacement versus anterior cervical fusion:

Data from four prospective, randomized, multicenter trials. Spine J 2011;11:S150–1.

7. Bhashyam N, De la Garza Ramos R, Nakhla J, et al. Thirty-day readmission and reoperation rates after single-level anterior cervical discectomy and fusion versus those after cervical disc replacement. Neurosurg Focus 2017;42:E6.

8. Jackson RJ, Davis RJ, Hoffman GA, et al. Subsequent surgery rates after cervical total disc replacement using a Mobi-C Cervical Disc Prosthesis versus anterior cervical discectomy and fusion: a prospective randomized clinical trial with 5-year follow-up. J Neurosurg Spine 2016;24:734–45.

9. Galbusera F, Bellini CM, Brayda-Bruno M, et al. Biomechanical studies on cervical total disc arthroplasty: A literature review. Clin Biomech (Bristol, Avon) 2008;23:1095–104.

10. Lou J, Li Y, Wang B, et al. In vitro biomechanical comparison after fixed- and mobile-core artificial cervical disc replacement versus fusion. Medicine (Baltimore) 2017;96:e8291.

11. Pham M, Phan K, Teng I, et al. Comparative study between M6-C and Mobi-C cervical artificial disc replacement: biomechanical outcomes and comparison with normative data. Orthop Surg 2018;10:84–8.

12. Wigfield C, Gill S, Nelson R, et al. Influence of an artificial cervical joint compared with fusion on adjacent-level motion in the treatment of degenerative cervical disc disease. J Neurosurg 2002;96:17–21.

13. Finn MA, Brodke DS, Daubs M, et al. Local and global subaxial cervical spine biomechanics after single-level fusion or cervical arthroplasty. Eur Spine J 2009;18:1520–7.

14. Guyer RD, Voronov LI, Havey RM, et al. Kinematic assessment of an elastic-core cervical disc prosthesis in one and two-level constructs. JOR Spine 2018;1:e1040.

15. Dmitriev AE, Cunningham BW, Hu N, et al. Adjacent level intradiscal pressure and segmental kinematics following a cervical total disc arthroplasty: an in vitro human cadaveric model. Spine 2005;30:1165–72.

16. Botolin S, Puttlitz C, Baldini T, et al. Facet joint biomechanics at the treated and adjacent levels after total disc replacement. Spine 2011;36:E27–32.

17. Kang H, Park P, La Marca F, et al. Analysis of load sharing on uncovertebral and facet joints at the C5-6 level with implantation of the Bryan, Prestige LP, or ProDisc-C cervical disc prosthesis: an in vivo image-based finite element study. Neurosurg Focus 2010;28:E9.

18. Link HD, McAfee PC, Pimenta L. Choosing a cervical disc replacement. Spine J 2004;4:294S–302S.

19. Huang RC, Girardi FP, Cammisa FP Jr, et al. The implications of constraint in lumbar total disc replacement. J Spinal Disord Tech 2003;16:412–7.

20. Sears WR, McCombe PF, Sasso RC. Kinematics of cervical and lumbar total disc replacement. Semin Spine Surg 2006;18:117–29.

21. Patwardhan AG, Havey RM. Biomechanics of cervical disc arthroplasty-A review of concepts and current technology. Int J Spine Surg 2020;14:S14–28.

22. Jacobs CAM, Siepe CJ, Ito K. Viscoelastic cervical total disc replacement devices: design concepts. Spine J 2020;20:1911–24.

23. Amadji M, Ameddah H, Mazouz H. Numerical study of the biomimetic M6-C Prosthesis with viscoelastic core. U.P.B Sci Bull, Series D 2019;81:121–34.

24. Patwardhan AG, Tzermiadianos MN, Tsitsopoulos PP, et al. Primary and coupled motions after cervical total disc replacement using a compressible six-degree-of-freedom prosthesis. Eur Spine J 2012;21:618–29.

25. Hui N, Phan K, Kerferd J, et al. Comparison of M6-C and Mobi-C cervical total disc replacement for cervical degenerative disc disease in adults. J Spine Surg 2019;5:393–403.

26. Lauryssen C, Coric D, Dimmig T, et al. Cervical total disc replacement using a novel compressible prosthesis: Results from a prospective FDA-regulated feasibility study with 24-month follow-up. Int J Spine Surg 2012;6:71–7.

27. Thomas S, Willems K, Van den Daelen L, et al. The M6-C cervical disc prosthesis: first clinical experience in 33 patients. Clin Spine Surg 2016;29:E182–7.

28. Byvaltsev VA, Kalinin AA, Stepanov IA, et al. Analysis of the results of total cervical disc arthroplasty using a M6-C prosthesis: a multicenter study. Zh Vopr Neirokhir Im N N Burdenko 2017;81:46–55.

29. Brenke C, Schmieder K, Barth M. Core herniation after implantation of a cervical artificial disc: case report. Eur Spine J 2015;24(Suppl 4):536–9.

30. Baltus C, Costa E, Vaz G, et al. Granulomatous reaction on a double-level cervical total disc arthroplasty: Case report. World Neurosurg 2019;122:360–3.

31. Harris L, Dyson E, Elliot M, et al. Delayed periprosthetic collection after cervical disc arthroplasty. J Neurosurg Spine 2019;1–8.

32. Xia MM, Winder MJ. M6-C cervical disc replacement failure associated with late onset infection. J Spine Surg 2019;5:584–8.

33. Chin KR, Pencle FJR, Seale JA, et al. Clinical outcomes of outpatient cervical total disc replacement compared with outpatient anterior cervical discectomy and fusion. Spine 2017;42:E567–74.

34. Chin KR, Lubinski JR, Zimmers KB, et al. Clinical experience and two-year follow-up with a one-piece viscoelastic cervical total disc replacement. J Spine Surg 2017;3:630–40.

35. Axiomed. Biocompatibility of the Freedom® Lumbar Disc and Freedom® Cervical Disc. Available at: https://static1.squarespace.com/static/5d079400cba6190001008b45/t/

5d138008e4b55100017995c3/1561559049065/ WPaperBiocomp.pdf 2012. downloaded 11-8-20.

36. Fransen P, Noriega D, Chatzisotiriou A, et al. One- or two- levels treatment by arthroplasty of cervical degenerative disease. Preliminary results after 5 years postoperative controls. J Spine 2018;7:1000405.

37. Reeks J, Liang H. Materials and their failure mechanisms in total disc replacement. Lubricants 2015;3:346–64.

38. Fransen P, Hansen-Algenstaedt N, Chatzisotiriou A, et al. Clinical results of cervical disc replacement with the Baguera C prosthesis after two years follow-up. Acta Orthop 2018;84:345–51.

39. Lee JH, Park WM, Kim YH, et al. A biomechanical analysis of an artificial disc with a shock-absorbing core property by using whole-cervical spine finite element analysis. Spine 2016;41:E893–901.

40. Maestretti G, Tropiano P, Fransen P, et al. Clinical and radiographic outcomes on a series of 249 patients treated with single and multilevel Baguera C Cervical Disc Replacement at 2-year follow up. International Society for the Advancement of Spine Surgery. Las Vegas, Nevada, April 26-30, 2011.

41. Heo DH, Lee DC, Oh JY, et al. Bone loss of vertebral bodies at the operative segment after cervical arthroplasty: a potential complication? Neurosurg Focus 2017;42:E7.

42. Kieser DC, Cawley DT, Fujishiro T, et al. Risk factors for anterior bone loss in cervical disc arthroplasty. J Neurosurg Spine 2018;29:123–9.

43. Sekhon LH, Duggal N, Lynch JJ, et al. Magnetic resonance imaging clarity of the Bryan, Prodisc-C, Prestige LP, and PCM cervical arthroplasty devices. Spine 2007;32:673–80.

44. Sundseth J, Jacobsen EA, Kolstad F, et al. Magnetic resonance imaging evaluation after implantation of a titanium cervical disc prosthesis: a comparison of 1.5 and 3 Tesla magnet strength. Eur Spine J 2013;22:2296–302.

45. Siskey R, Ciccarelli L, Lui MK, et al. Are PEEK-on-ceramic bearings an option for total disc arthroplasty? An in vitro tribology study. Clin Orthop Relat Res 2016;474:2428–40.

46. Xin H, Shepherd DET, Dearn KD. A tribological assessment of a PEEK based self-mating total cervical disc replacement. Wear 2013;303:473–9.

47. Xin H, Shepherd D, Dearn K. PEEK (Polyether-etherketone) based cervical total disc arthroplasty: Contact stress and lubrication analysis. Open Biomed Eng J 2012;6:73–9.

48. Shibayama M, Ito F, Miura Y, et al. Early results of the NuNec cervical disc replacement. International Society for the Advancement of Spine Surgery. Las Vegas, Nevada, April, 26-30, 2011.

49. Turner I, Choi D. NuNec™ Cervical Disc Arthroplasty improves quality of life in cervical radiculopathy and myelopathy: A 2-yr follow-up. Neurosurgery 2018; 83:422–8.

50. Lazaro BC, Yucesoy K, Yuksel KZ, et al. Effect of arthroplasty design on cervical spine kinematics: analysis of the Bryan Disc, ProDisc-C, and Synergy Disc. Neurosurg Focus 2010;28:E6.

51. Yücesoy K, Yüksel KZ, Yüksel M, et al. Changes in sagittal alignment after cervical disc arthroplasty: results of 24-month-pilot study. J Nervous Sys Surg 2016;6:1–9.

52. Yucesoy K, Yuksel KZ, Altun I, et al. Can cervical arthroplasty impact alignment? A comparison of the Synergy Disc with cervical fusion. J Spine 2017;6: 1000400.

53. Havey RM, Khayatzadeh S, Voronov LI, et al. Motion response of a polycrystalline diamond adaptive axis of rotation cervical total disc arthroplasty. Clin Biomech (Bristol, Avon) 2019;62:34–41.

54. McNally D, Naylor J, Johnson S. An in vitro biomechanical comparison of Cadisc™-L with natural lumbar discs in axial compression and sagittal flexion. Eur Spine J 2012;21(Suppl 5):S612–7.

55. Mahomed A, Moghadas PM, Shepherd DE, et al. Effect of axial load on the flexural properties of an elastomeric total disc replacement. Spine 2012;37:E908–12.

56. Grassner L, Grillhosl A, Bierschneider M, et al. Disc herniation caused by a viscoelastic nucleus after total lumbar disc replacement-a case report. J Spine Surg 2018;4:478–82.

57. Fuentes S, Metellus P. Metal free cervical disc prosthesis: First clinical results and MRI compatiblity. International Society for the Advancement of Spine Surgery. Vancouver, Canada, April 3-5, 2013.

58. Kienle A, Graf N, Krais C, et al. The MOVE-C Cervical Artificial Disc - Design, materials, mechanical safety. Med Devices (Auckl) 2020;13:315–24.

59. Dong L, Tan MS, Yan QH, et al. Footprint mismatch of cervical disc prostheses with Chinese cervical anatomic dimensions. Chin Med J (Engl) 2015;128: 197–202.

60. Thaler M, Hartmann S, Gstottner M, et al. Footprint mismatch in total cervical disc arthroplasty. Eur Spine J 2013;22:759–65.

Cervical Total Disc Replacement
Long-Term Outcomes

Gregory Callanan, DO[a],*, Kristen E. Radcliff, MD[b]

KEYWORDS

• Cervical disc arthroplasty • Disc replacement • Anterior cervical discectomy and fusion (ACDF)
• Radiculopathy • Myelopathy • Cervical degenerative disc disease

KEY POINTS

- Degenerative disc disease and associated cervical spondylosis are common disorders encountered in clinical practice that may cause progressive cervical radicular or myelopathic symptoms.
- Surgical management has historically consisted of removal of pathologic disc material, decompression of neural elements, and interspace fusion.
- Cervical total disc arthroplasty has emerged as an alternative procedure to avoid several potential complications of arthrodesis, including loss of cervical range of motion with potential effects with respect to adjacent segment degeneration and disease, pseudoarthrosis, and complications regarding intervertebral graft.
- This article discusses recent literature regarding long-term outcomes of total disc arthroplasty in detail.
- Cervical total disc arthroplasty is a safe and effective surgical alternative in properly selected patients with cervical radiculopathy and myelopathy.

BACKGROUND

Disorder of the cervical spine is a common clinical problem encountered by physicians. The cervical spine is composed of 7 vertebrae. The subaxial cervical spine is defined as C3 to C7 vertebral levels. The vertebral bodies are mobile structures that are connected via cartilaginous intervertebral discs. An intervertebral disc consists of an outer annulus fibrosis and a central nucleus pulposus. The spine plays an important role in protecting and housing the spinal cord and associated nerve roots.

Progressive wear and tear of these intervertebral discs resulting in degenerative disc disease often leads to the progression of cervical spondylosis or spinal stenosis. These changes can cause cervical radicular or myelopathic symptoms,

which can lead to significant impairment to patients. Surgical management has consisted of removal of pathologic disc material, decompression of neurologic structures, and interspace fusion.

Anterior cervical discectomy and fusion (ACDF) has been a reliable and often-used surgical treatment of cervical myelopathy and radiculopathy with long-term clinical success.[1,2] Performing a successful ACDF consists of removal of pathologic disc material, decompression of neurologic elements, restoration of disc height via intervertebral graft, and segmental stabilization by plating to improve fusion rate. The use of an anterior cervical plate has also been shown to reduce the incidence of pseudarthrosis for multilevel fusions while simultaneously maintaining sagittal balance.[3]

[a] Department of Orthopedic Surgery, Inspira Health Network, Vineland, NJ 08360, USA; [b] Department of Orthopedic Surgery, Thomas Jefferson University, Rothman Institute, 2500 English Creek Avenue, Egg Harbor Township, NJ 08234, USA
* Corresponding author.
E-mail address: callanang@ihn.org

Neurosurg Clin N Am 32 (2021) 461–472
https://doi.org/10.1016/j.nec.2021.05.007
1042-3680/21/

Although ACDF has proved itself as an effective surgical treatment option for cervical myelopathy and radiculopathy, it has its own set of potential complications. The limitations of ACDF include loss of cervical range of motion (ROM), the concern for adjacent segment degeneration (ASD) and disease, pseudarthrosis, complications related to the choice of intervertebral graft, dysphagia, as well as standard anterior cervical approach risks.

Although decompression and fusion of the symptomatic level may provide relief, it may have deleterious biomechanical effects on the surrounding segments. Arthrodesis at a specific segment can lead to increased stress at adjacent segment discs above and below the construct, thereby leading to accelerated degeneration. The radiographic finding consistent with degeneration adjacent to the construct is known as ASD. The clinical manifestations and symptoms associated with these degenerative changes are known as ASD.

Hilibrand and colleagues[4] reported an annual incidence of adjacent segment disease of 2.9% per year in 374 patients after ACDF. In the decade following this procedure, they estimated that approximately 25% of patients who undergo cervical fusion develop ASD, of whom two-thirds proceed to require subsequent surgical interventions. However, within the same study, the risk of new disease at an adjacent level was significantly lower following multilevel fusion compared with single-level arthrodesis, suggesting that symptomatic adjacent segment disease is the result of progressive spondylosis.

Goffin and colleagues[2] reported that the rate of radiographic degeneration of adjacent segments following arthrodesis was 60% over 5 years for traumatic cervical injuries. The similarities noted in this study between their cohort of younger patients with trauma and older atraumatic patients suggest that both the biomechanical impact of the interbody fusion and the natural progression of prior degenerative disease act as triggering factors for ASD.[2]

Pseudarthrosis is another concern regarding fusion. Pseudarthrosis is described as failure of fusion at 1 year. The rates of pseudarthrosis for single-level arthrodesis ranges from 3% to 20% and 21% to 46% for 2-level and 3-level fusions respectively.[5,6] There are several factors that can contribute to fusion rates, including graft selection, patient comorbidities, surgical technique, and the number of levels involved.

There has been an effort in the academic community to investigate the various choices of bone graft in order to improve fusion rates following ACDF. Iliac crest bone graft (ICBG) was historically considered the gold standard for use in ACDF.[7] However, there are numerous donor site issues reported with the use of ICBG, including persistent pain, difficulty with ambulation, and numbness. Other issues associated with autograft harvest of ICBG include infection risk, wound healing complications, potential soft tissue herniation through the donor site, and hematomas with reported complication rates of 10% to 39%.[8,9]

Allograft use removes the need for harvesting graft and therefore the associated complications as well. However, allograft use can have complications. There have been reports in the literature of bioincompatibility and disease transmission. Because of these factors, there remains a high interest in bone graft substitutes using demineralized bone matrix, ceramic-based bone grafts, and nanofiber-based collagen scaffolds.[10,11]

Cervical total disc arthroplasty (TDA) has emerged as another operative procedure as an alternative to ACDF in order to avoid the aforementioned complications associated with arthrodesis. There are no pseudarthrosis risks given the nature of the procedure, nor any issues pertaining to allograft or autograft bone graft. The goal is to prevent ASD and maintain ROM at the vertebral segment.

HISTORY OF TOTAL DISC ARTHROPLASTY

The goal of TDA is to alleviate the symptoms the patient is experiencing while providing a biomechanically efficient, stable, and safe construct. There are certain anatomic characteristics unique to the cervical spine that must be taken into consideration regarding TDA design in order for successful patient outcomes. One such consideration is the limited bone stock available in the cervical spine, resulting in less flexibility when performing bony cuts for accommodation of the implant. In addition, the intervertebral discs play an essential role in maintaining balance of the middle and anterior columns, thereby providing spinal stability. Compared with lower extremity arthroplasty, most TDA candidates are typically younger. This longer lifespan corresponds to an estimated 100 million flexion cycles for a given implant.[8] This concern for wear debris and potential inflammatory reaction are of concern given the close proximity of the implant to the spinal cord and structures of the anterior neck and are currently under investigation.

The earliest application of TDA was in the United Kingdom in the 1980s by Cummins and colleagues[12] The device developed and used was a metal-on-metal ball-and-socket construct. Since then, newer materials and fixation methods have been developed for implantation in the cervical spine. The Cervical Spine Study group developed a nomenclature system for cervical arthroplasty.[13] Arthroplasty implants are characterized by material, articulation, fixation, design, and kinematics. They can be classified as nonarticulating, articulating, or biarticulating. Various designs include metal-on-metal (Prestige ST and LP; Medtronic Sofamor Danek, Memphis, TN), metal-on-polymer (Bryan, Medtronic Sofamor Danek; ProDisc-C, Synthes Spine, West Chester, PA; Mobi-C, LDR Medical Tryoes, France), ceramic-on-polymer, or ceramic-on-ceramic implants. Discs may be nonmodular (nonreplaceable components) or modular (with replaceable parts). Further classification with respect to motion are noted as constrained, semiconstrained, or unconstrained. Unconstrained devices rely on soft tissue and the inherent compression across the intervertebral disc space in order to limit motion, semiconstrained devices allow for physiologic motion, and constrained devices restrict motion to that less than physiologic.

BIOMECHANICS

The biomechanical goals of TDA include restoration of physiologic kinematics and mobility while maintaining spinal stability, protection of biological structures from overloading, and device stability and response to wear debris.[14] Biomechanically, the most researched parameter concerning TDA is ROM. There have been several ex vivo studies investigating ROM following TDA that have shown overall motion preservation at the index level similar to physiologic ROM irrespective of prosthesis design.[15–17]

During flexion and extension, normal cervical spine movement shows anteroposterior (AP) translation. The cervical spinal motion segment consists of the disc and 2 facets. Disc prosthesis design must take into consideration these 3 compartments in conjunction with the multiple ligamentous structures of the cervical spine for motion preservation.

Biomechanical investigations have indicated that the semiconstrained design (ball-in-trough design) of the Prestige cervical disc permits normal kinematics within all ROMs. With respect to constrained designs (ball-in-socket designs), DiAngelo and colleagues[15] reported that a constrained design failed to reproduce normal motion in extension. The constrained design does not allow the physiologic AP translation that occurs with normal facet joint motion. A balance of all the significant structures within the cervical spine, including the ligaments and facets, is essential

because of their complex relationship with respect to normal cervical spine movement.

This balancing act becomes even more apparent with extension. During cervical flexion, the unshingling of the facets diminishes their involvement in constraining the motion of the functional spine unit. However, with extension, the facets shingle, thereby becoming more involved with motion constraint. With both a constrained facet joint and constrained disc joint, it would be expected to have limited motion because of the effects of 1 joint working against the other, which may result in decreased motion or increased stress on the system.

Sasso and colleagues[18] performed a prospective, randomized, multicenter clinical trial to study kinematic analysis of target-level and adjacent motion segments. Patients underwent single-level arthrodesis (Atlantis anterior cervical plate, n = 221) or single-level arthroplasty (Bryan cervical disc prosthesis, n = 242) at C3 to C7. Patients underwent neutral, flexion, and extension lateral radiographs preoperatively and at regular intervals for 2 years. Researchers noted that significantly more motion was retained within the arthroplasty group compared with the arthrodesis group at the index level. The arthroplasty group on average retained 7.95° at 24 months. The preoperative motion was 6.43° without evidence of degradation over 2 years. This finding is in contrast with the motion in the arthrodesis group, which was 1.1° at 3-month follow-up and gradually diminished to 0.87° at 2 years. The preoperative motion was 8.39°. In addition, there were no cases of subsidence or migration at 2 years with the Bryan disc. In addition, there was no evidence of bridging bone heterotopic ossification (HO) within the arthroplasty group.

Gandhi and colleagues[19] performed a cadaveric biomechanical study comparing arthroplasty with arthrodesis using human cadaveric spines. The investigators took 11 specimens (C2–T1) which were divided into 2 groups (Bryan and Prestige LP). The specimens were tested in the following order: intact, single-level total disc replacement (TDR) at C5-C6 level, 2-level TDR at C5-C6-C7 levels, fusion at C5-C6 level and TDR at C6-C7 level (hybrid construct), and a 2-level fusion. The intact specimens were tested up to a moment of 2.0 Nm. After every surgical intervention, the constructs were loaded until the primary motion (C2–T1) matched the motion of the respective intact state (hybrid control). They found that cervical disc arthroplasty with both the Bryan and Prestige LP discs not only preserved motion at the operated level but also maintained normal motion at the adjacent levels. Under simulated physiologic loading, the motion patterns of the cervical spine after arthroplasty were very similar to the intact motion pattern compared with fusion. Furthermore, their results suggested that an adjacent segment disc arthroplasty was more favorable from a biomechanical perspective compared with a fusion in the presence of a preexisting fusion.

INDICATIONS AND CONTRAINDICATIONS OF TOTAL DISC ARTHROPLASTY

At this time, the US Food and Drug Administration (FDA)–approved indications for cervical disc arthroplasty are single-level and dual-level cervical degenerative disc disease causing radiculopathy and/or myelopathy in adult patients.[20] Patients should exhaust conservative management modalities before discussion of operative interventions. Disc herniation and foraminal osteophytes causing radiculopathy or disc herniation causing myelopathy are both additional indications for TDA. With regard to cervical disc arthroplasty in patients with myelopathy, there was a concern regarding the preservation of cervical motion potentially maintaining microtrauma to the spinal cord. Riew and colleagues[21] showed that patients with single-level disease, and patients treated with arthroplasty for an abnormality localized to the disc space compared with arthrodesis showed similar clinical improvement as measured via Nurick grade, neck disability index (NDI), 36-Item Short-Form Health Survey (SF-36) scores, and visual analog scale (VAS) at 2 years postoperatively.[21] However, this study did not evaluate the treatment of retrovertebral compression as occurs in ossification of the posterior longitudinal ligament, congenital stenosis, or ligamentum flavum hypertrophy.

Proper patient selection for TDA is paramount to successful patient outcomes. Contraindications to the procedure include osteoporosis or metabolic bone disease, facet arthritis, ankylosis, active or prior infection, congenital cervical stenosis, and segmental cervical instability. In addition, arthroplasty requires the dorsal elements to be both intact and functional because these posterior elements are essential to prosthesis stability; therefore, prior laminectomy or excessive facet removal are contraindications to TDA. Additional relative contraindications include rheumatoid arthritis, renal failure, cancer, preoperative corticosteroid medication, ossification of the posterior longitudinal ligament, and diffuse idiopathic skeletal hyperostosis.[22]

COMPLICATIONS

Complications following TDA can be related to several factors, including patient selection,

surgical technique, or the prosthesis itself. Proper patient selection is essential to avoiding complications during TDA. Patients with sagittal deformity, facet arthropathy, osteoporosis, metabolic bone disease, preoperative instability, or previous dorsal cervical surgery are not preferable candidates for TDA and arthroplasty should be avoided in these patients.

Although arthroplasty procedures inherently do not have a risk of pseudarthrosis or graft donor site morbidity, patients undergoing TDA are still susceptible to the same anterior cervical approach–related complications as arthrodesis, including dysphagia, voice hoarseness, vascular injury, neurologic injury, and hematoma.[23,24]

Cervical positioning before surgery to ensure proper alignment is critical given that cervical arthroplasty is not designed for correction of sagittal deformity.[25,26] A slightly lordotic to neutral cervical alignment is preferred. Correct implant sizing is also paramount to TDA success. Implants that are not large enough may migrate with repetitive motion, whereas implants that are too large can hinder ROM.

Implant subsidence or migration is also of concern with arthroplasty procedures. This problem may manifest as postoperative cervical alignment changes or potentially as new-onset neurologic complaints.[27] Inadequate end-plate preparation could be a contributing factor to this complication. Of note, patients with metabolic bone disease or osteoporosis may undergo implant subsidence regardless of adequate end-plate preparation or proper implant sizing.

HO is a unique complication noted after cervical arthroplasty. HO is the formation of bone outside of skeletal bony elements. The proposed mechanism of HO involves differentiation of mesenchymal cells originating from bone or muscle to osteoblasts, which are capable of spreading into the peripheral soft tissue and vasculature. The osteogenic agents that are released from tissues attached to bone are often the result of local intraoperative injury.[28] It has been noted that HO occurs early in the postoperative period and may be present in 34% of patients at 4 years and 38% of patients at 6 years.[29] Thorough and gratuitous use of irrigation intraoperatively and limited muscle retraction have been advocated to help minimize the formation and risk of HO. In addition, the early use of postoperative nonsteroidal antiinflammatory drugs is reported to help decrease both the severity and incidence of HO.

Vertebral fracture is another potential complication during TDA. Although this complication may arise with any TDA device, there have been several reports described in the literature of this occurring with implantation of keeled-type implants.[16,30,31] The bony preparation required with the keeled-type implants may lead to fracture in osteoporotic patients or those with otherwise diminished bone quality. There is increased concern when performing dual-level TDA using keeled implants because this creates 2 central keel cuts within the same vertebral body, which may potentially lead to fracture.[32] Moreover, osteolysis secondary to inflammatory response to the implant may weaken the vertebral body, which can potentially lead to fracture.

SURGICAL TECHNIQUE

It is important to have a discussion with the patient before performing TDA regarding the potential need to make an intraoperative decision, if at any point during the surgery it becomes evident that arthroplasty is contraindicated, to perform an arthrodesis alternative.

Patient positioning for an arthroplasty procedure should have the cervical spine preferably physiologic or placed in slightly lordotic alignment. Underneath the neck, a small towel roll may be positioned in order to assist with proper positioning of the cervical spine while avoiding hyperlordosis. The head may be supported on a pillow or carefully positioned towels to maintain stability throughout the procedure. The benefit of improved intraoperative visualization should be weighed against the risks of traction injury when considering a taping technique of the shoulders.

A Smith-Robinson approach to the cervical spine is performed with appropriate localization of the segment. After adequate decompression is performed at the affected level, disc arthroplasty is performed. The surgeon should take careful note to perform extensive hemostasis throughout the procedure to minimize blood loss but also to decrease the risk of HO. Before end-plate preparation, it is imperative to ensure the proper position of the vertebrae in both the sagittal and coronal plane via fluoroscopic imaging. End plates are prepared according to the device to be implanted. It is very important to preserve subchondral bone while preparing the end plates in order to minimize the risk of implant subsidence.

After appropriate confirmation of adequate neurologic decompression, vertebral alignment, and end plate preparation, implantation of an appropriately sized implant may be performed. When satisfied with implant position, it may be secured to the spine via implant-specific instrumentation.

With the implant secured, final imaging may be performed before wound closure. Confirmation of hemostasis should be performed and wound closure may be performed in typical standard fashion. Postoperative immobilization is not required. Standing flexion and extension radiograph images should be obtained before discharge to serve as a reference and comparison for follow-up purposes.

CLINICAL EVIDENCE
Prestige Disc

The Prestige ST arthroplasty construct is a ball-and-trough design composed of stainless steel containing iron, carbon, nickel, molybdenum, and chromium. This device uses dual-screw fixation to each respective adjacent vertebral body with thin anterior flanges.

In 2007, the 2-year data from a prospective, randomized, multicenter study analyzing the results of cervical TDA (Prestige ST) compared with ACDF in patients treated for symptomatic single-level cervical degenerative disc disease were published.[20] The investigators reported that the Prestige ST cervical disc system maintained physiologic segmental motion at 2 years after implantation and was associated with improved neurologic success, improved clinical outcomes, and a reduced rate of secondary surgeries compared with arthrodesis.

Five-year data were published by Burkus and colleagues[33] in 2010 regarding the previously mentioned FDA investigational device exemption (IDE) clinical trial. Researchers reported significant improvements in NDI, SF-36 scores, and Neck and Arm Pain Numerical Rating Scale scores in both groups by 1.5 months, which were sustained at 5 years.[33] The arthroplasty group experienced a significantly greater mean NDI improvement score at 3 and 5 years compared with the arthrodesis group. The arthroplasty implant also maintained angular motion effectively with more than 7.3° on average at 3 years and 6.5° at 5 years after surgery. No cases of implant migration were observed up to 60 months. Reoperation rates were significantly different between the two groups with 0% of arthroplasty group compared with 1.9% of the arthrodesis group.

The Prestige LP artificial disc is composed of a titanium and ceramic composite with rails to act as migratory prevention through friction and a plasma spray coating on both inferior and superior surfaces to help encourage bony ingrowth.[26] Gornet and colleagues[34] published a prospective, multicenter IDE study in 2015. These researchers prospectively collected Prestige LP data from 20 investigational sites, which were compared with data from 265 historical control arthrodesis patients from the initial Prestige ST IDE study. Clinical outcomes measured included SF-36, NDI, Neck and Arm Pain Numerical Rating Scale, work status, disc height, ROM, adverse events, additional procedures, and neurologic status. Clinical and radiographic evaluations were completed preoperatively, intraoperatively, and at 1.5, 3, 6, 12, and 24 months postoperatively. This study noted significant improvements in NDI, neck/arm pain, SF-36, and neurologic status in both the Prestige LP and arthrodesis group by 1.5 months, which were maintained at 2 years postoperatively. The median return-to-work time for the arthroplasty group was 40 days compared with 60 days for the arthrodesis group. The mean angular motion following implantation of the Prestige LP device was maintained at 1 year (7.9°) and 2 years (7.5°). The investigators reported that this device maintains mean postoperative segmental motion while providing the potential for biomechanical stability with significantly improved clinical outcomes compared with baseline, at least noninferior to ACDF, up to 24 months after surgery.

Gornet and colleagues[35] in 2019 published the 10-year outcomes of the Prestige LP cervical disc arthroplasty compared with ACDF for treatment of degenerative cervical spine disease at 2 adjacent levels. This prospective, randomized controlled, multicenter FDA IDE had 209 patients receive arthroplasty procedure at 2 levels compared with 188 patients who underwent ACDF. Ten-year follow-up data were available for 148 TDA and 118 ACDF patients. Clinical and radiographic evaluations were completed preoperatively, intraoperatively, and postoperatively. From 2 to 10 years, TDA was superior statistically with regard to overall success compared with arthrodesis, with rates at 10 years of 80.4% versus 62.2% respectively. The investigators also noted that improvements from preoperative results in NDI and neck pain scores were significantly greater in the TDA group compared with arthrodesis. The TDA group also experienced statistically fewer secondary surgical interventions at the index level (4.7%) compared with the arthrodesis group (17.6%). The TDA group also experienced statistically fewer secondary surgical interventions at the adjacent levels as well (9% compared with 17.9%).

Bryan Disc

The Bryan prosthetic disc is a semiconstrained, biarticulating device that consists of 3 components. There are 2 titanium alloy end plates, which have a porous surface to promote bony ingrowth and stability, as well as a polyurethane center. There is an anterior flange on these end points to act as stop points to help prevent posterior dislocation of the device into the canal. The polyurethane core is noted to be enclosed by a saline-filled sheath, which becomes a pseudocapsule over time. The goal of this pseudocapsule is the replication of the natural vertebral discs' cushioning effect.[36]

In 2009, Heller and colleagues[37] published a comparison of Bryan cervical disc arthroplasty with ACDF as part of the FDA IDE trial. This prospective, randomized, multicenter clinical trial had 242 patients treated with arthroplasty, whereas the control group included 221 patients who underwent single-level ACDF. Patients underwent radiographs and clinical examinations at regular intervals for 2 years postoperatively. Analysis of 1-year and 2-year postoperative data showed improvement in all clinical outcome measures for both groups, including NDI, SF-36, as well as numerical rating scales for neck and arm pain. There was a significantly greater improvement in the arthroplasty group with respect to NDI, neck pain, return to work, and overall success.

In 2011, the 4-year clinical data on 181 patients who received the Bryan disc and 138 patients who underwent ACDF were reported.[38] Substantial reduction in NDI occurred in both groups compared with preoperative values. The greater improvement in NDI score in the Bryan disc cohort persisted throughout the 48-month follow-up period. The improvement in arm pain score was substantial for both groups but was significantly higher in the Bryan disc group, as was the case regarding SF-36 scores. The mean ROM for the Bryan disc was 8.08° and 8.48° at 24 and 48 months respectively. Total and serious adverse event rates were similar across both groups. The 4-year overall success rates were 81.5% and 72.5% for the arthroplasty and fusion groups respectively, which was statistically significant.

Zhao and colleagues[39] published their 10-year long-term outcomes for the Bryan prosthetic disc device and reported improvement in patients with myelopathy using the modified Japanese Orthopaedic Association (mJOA) score. The investigators also noted improvement in patients' radicular symptoms based on NDI and VAS. ROM at the operated level was baseline 7.8° and diminished to 4.7° at final follow-up. ASD was noted in 47.6% of operated levels. No patient was noted to have adjacent segment disease. HO was noted in 69% of operated levels; however, only 2 patients developed recurrent radiculopathy as a result requiring operative interventions.

ProDisc-C

The ProDisc-C prosthetic disc is a ball-and-socket, 2-piece, semiconstrained device. The porous end plates consist of cobalt chrome alloy. Attached to the internal surface of the inferior end plate is a convex ultrahigh-molecular-weight insert. This insert articulates with the inner surface of the superior end plate, which is concave. Translation is limited with this design, but rotation is permitted within all 3 axes. The superior and inferior external surfaces of the implant end plates are coated with titanium plasma spray and possess slotted keels.[40]

Murrey and colleagues[41] published the results of the prospective, randomized controlled, multicenter FDA IDE study of the ProDisc-C TDA versus ACDF for the treatment of 1-level symptomatic cervical disc disease. This study was conducted at 13 sites with 209 patients randomized and treated (106 ACDF; 103 ProDisc-C). VAS pain and intensity (neck and arm), NDI, neurologic examination, device success, adverse event occurrence, and SF-36 were measured. Patients were assessed preoperatively and postoperatively at 6 weeks and 3, 6, 12, 18, and 24 months. Both groups showed significant improvement from baseline; however, there was no statistically significant improvement between the two groups at 2 years. There was a statistically significant difference in the number of secondary surgeries, with 8.5% of arthrodesis patients requiring a secondary surgery within the 2-year postoperative period compared with 1.8% of the ProDisc-C patients. At 2 years, there was also a statistically significant difference between medication usage, with 89.9% of ProDisc-C patients not using strong narcotics or muscle relaxants, in contrast with 81.5% of arthrodesis patients.

Zigler and colleagues[42] published the 5-year clinical data for the ProDisc FDA IDE. Patients had statistically significant diminished neck pain intensity and frequency compared with arthrodesis group. They reported no failures of the device or implant migration 5 years postoperatively. It was also noted that ProDisc-C patients underwent reoperation at a significantly lower rate compared with arthrodesis group (2.9% compared with 11.3% respectively).

Kelly and colleagues[43] compared adjacent segment motion following ACDF versus ProDisc-C TDA. This study did not show a significant difference in adjacent segment ROM between ACDF and TDA. The investigators concluded that further clinical follow-up is needed to determine whether possible differences in adjacent segment motion influence the prevalence of adjacent segment disease between the two groups.

Mobi-C

The Mobi-C prosthetic disc is composed of 3 individual components. The 2 end plates are composed of cobalt, chromium, 29 molybdenum ISO 5832-12 alloy coated with titanium and hydroxyapatite spray. These end plates are each lined with teeth on the lateral edge of their external surfaces. The internal contact surface of the inferior end plate is spherical and the superior end plate is flat. The core centers itself on the inferior plate while it is laterally inhibited by 2 stops, and continuously recenters itself while the superior plate moves, allowing for translational and rotational motion.[44]

The Mobi-C cervical disc was the first cervical disc arthroplasty with FDA approval for usage in 2-level cervical disc arthroplasty.[45] Kim and colleagues[45] published their data from a retrospective study with 23 patients who underwent single-level TDA with the Mobi-C disc prosthesis. The investigators reported a statistically significant improvement with respect to VAS arm and neck pain scores at 6-month follow-up. Also of note, patients returned to work within 1 month postoperatively. No complications were reported within this study. Further investigation comparing Mobi-C TDA with ACDF was performed by Park and colleagues,[46] who published their findings in 2008. They evaluated 53 patients treated for cervical disc herniations with radiculopathy. Twenty-one patients underwent arthroplasty with Mobi-C and 32 patients underwent ACDF. Clinical outcomes measured included VAS, NDI, duration of hospital stay, and convalesce time.[46] There were significantly shorter hospital stays and quicker return-to-work times in the TDA group compared with the arthrodesis group. Both NDI and extremity VAS score improved in 12 months for both groups. In addition, no complications were noted within the TDA group; however, there were 5 cage subsidence events within the arthrodesis group.

Guerin and colleagues[47] analyzed the sagittal balance after single-level TDA using Mobi-C disc prosthesis. This prospective study analyzed the sagittal balance in 40 patients in addition to measuring the clinical outcomes of these patients via SF-36, NDI, and VAS. This study showed maintenance of sagittal alignment, cervical lordosis, and cervical ROM 2 years postoperatively. In addition, they also showed significant improvement of SF-36, NDI, and VAS for the arthroplasty group. Beaurain and colleagues[48] also reported clinical and radiological results of cervical TDR with 2-year follow-up. Seventy-six patients who underwent Mobi-C TDA had clinical and radiographic data collected throughout 24 months. This study showed significant improvements in VAS arm and neck pain indices, SF-36, and NDI scores. Motion was preserved over the time at index levels with a mean ROM of 9° at 2 years postoperatively. The investigators also recorded no instances of subsidence or migration of implant.

With respect to 2-level arthroplasty, Davis and colleagues[49] published their results comparing Mobi-C TDA with arthrodesis for 2-level contiguous cervical degenerative disc disease with 2-year follow-up. In this prospective, multicenter, randomized FDA IDE, 205 patients received the Mobi-C TDR device and 105 patients underwent ACDF. On average, both groups experienced significant improvements in NDI and VAS neck and arm pain score from baseline. Of note, the TDA group experienced significantly greater improvement in NDI at all time points; VAS neck pain score at 6 weeks; and at 3, 6, and 12 months postoperatively. The reoperation rate was also significantly higher in the ACDF group at 11.4% compared with 3.1% for the TDA group.

Radcliff and colleagues[50] published their 7-year data from a continuation of the prospective, multicenter, randomized FDA IDE clinical trial comparing Mobi-C TDA with ACDF. Outcome measure were recorded both preoperatively and postoperatively at 6 weeks and subsequently at 3, 6, 12, 18 months, and annually through 60 months, and at 84 months. Outcomes measured included NDI, VAS neck and arm pain, segmental ROM, patient satisfaction, SF-12 Mental Composite Score (MCS)/Physical Composite Score (PCS), major complications, overall success, and subsequent surgery rate. With respect to TDA, 164 patients were treated with single-level TDA and 225 patients were treated with 2-level TDA. The ACDF group had 81 patients treated with single-level ACDF and 105 patients treated with 2-level ACDF. At 7 years, follow-up rates ranged from 73.5% to 84.4% (overall 80.2%). The overall success rates of 2-level TDA and ACDF were 60.8% and 34.2% respectively. The overall success rates for single-level TDA and ACDF were 55.2% and 50% respectively. Both the TDA and ACDF groups experienced significant improvement in baseline NDI scores, SF-12 MCS/PCS scores, and VAS neck and arm pain scores. In both the single-level and 2-level TDA cohorts, a significantly higher percentage of patients rated themselves as very satisfied with their treatment compared with the ACDF group (90.9% and 85.9% compared with 77.8% and 73.9% respectively). The rate of adjacent level secondary surgery was significantly lower in both the single-level and 2-level TDA group compared with ACDF (3.7% and 4.4% compared with

13.6% and 11.3% respectively). Their study showed the clinical superiority of 2-level TDA compared with ACDF and noninferiority of single-level TDA compared with ACDF.[50]

DISCOVER

The Discover prosthetic disc is a ball-and-socket prosthesis. It is composed of 2 titanium alloy end plates with an ultrahigh-molecular-weight polyethylene center. It is an unconstrained prosthesis. The titanium alloy end plates are coated with porous titanium spray and hydroxyapatite. The end plates are lined with 1-mm teeth to allow immediate fixation. The spherical bearing allows motion in all rotational directions.[51]

Li and colleagues[51] published their study reporting the clinical outcomes following TDA using the Discover prosthetic disc. Fifty-five patients were prospectively followed for 2 years and outcome measurements, including JOA, NDI, and VAS, were recorded. Mean NDI, JOA, and VAS scores showed statistically significant improvements at last follow-up. Anterior migration of prosthesis was noted in 6 patients. HO was noted to occur in 10 patients. The investigators additionally reported that postoperative functional spinal unit (FSU) motion positively correlated with preoperative FSU motion.

Skeppholm and colleagues[52] published their 2-year FDA IDE prospective randomized clinical trial data investigating the Discover prosthetic disc compared with ACDF and reported that both procedures provided statistically significant decreases in NDI. No significant statistical differences were noted between arthroplasty or fusion in this study with respect to NDI, VAS, or health-related quality of life as measured by EQ-5D.

CerviCore

The CerviCore prosthetic device is a 2-piece semi-constrained design. The device is made of cobalt-chromium-molybdenum. This device has a saddle bearing design that permits 2 independent centers of rotation, 1 for flexion/extension and 1 for lateral bending. An anterior stop is built into the device to prevent posterior dislocation into the canal. The external surface of each base is coated with titanium plasma spray and contains 2 fins, each of which contains 3 spikes.[53]

A cadaveric study compared the CerviCore with arthrodesis with respect to ROM. The investigators noted that, with respect to ROM, the CerviCore group experienced deviations from intact biomechanics less substantially compared with after fusion.[54]

Secure-C

The Secure-C prosthetic disc is a semiconstrained device consisting of 3 components. The device consists of 2 keeled porous spray–coated cobalt chrome alloy end plates with an ultrahigh-molecular-weight polyethylene sliding center. The superior surface of the center piece is spherical and the inferior piece is cylindrical, which allows for AP sliding, allowing more physiologic loading and a moving instantaneous axis of rotation in the sagittal plane. This design eliminates dislodgement of the core, helping to protect facets from excess loading.[55]

Vaccaro and colleagues[56] published 2-year results from a randomized, prospective, multicenter FDA IDE clinical trial comparing Secure-C. A total of 380 patients from 18 investigational sites were prospectively enrolled in the study. Patients were evaluated postoperatively at 6 weeks and 3, 6, 12, and 24 months. Clinical outcomes were recorded, including overall success, VAS neck and arm, NDI, neurologic status, SF-36, ROM, and adverse events. The investigators reported superiority in overall success and patient satisfaction at 24 months comparing SECURE-C with ACDF. In addition, the SECURE-C group also showed noninferiority compared with arthrodesis with respect to NDI, VAS neck and arm scores, and neurologic status.

M6

The M6 prosthetic disc is a single-piece device with titanium alloy end plates and a complex center piece. The center piece is polycarbonate urethane polymeric material. This material acts as the nucleus pulposus, which is surrounded by a polyethylene woven fiber construct that serves as the annulus fibrosis. A polymer sheath surrounds the center piece, thereby preventing entry of debris or ingrowth of tissues. The external surface of each end plate has 3 keels present. The external surfaces are coated with porous titanium.[57]

Reyes-Sanchez and colleagues[58] reported their results for 25 patients treated with the M6 artificial disc, which showed a significant decrease in NDI scores. This improvement was more pronounced in single-level patients compared with 2-level patients. In addition, patients with a shorter duration of symptoms were also noted to have more pronounced improvement of NDI scores. A similar result was noted with respect to neck and arm pain. By 24 months, the mean ROM value at the operated level had returned to approximately the preoperative ROM. No serious device-related adverse events, repeat operative interventions, or radiographic evidence of HO or migration were noted.

FUTURE CONSIDERATIONS

Much of the recent literature regarding cervical disc arthroplasty, regardless of the specific device, has sought to show not only noninferiority of arthroplasty compared with arthrodesis also that arthroplasty decreases the incidence of ASD in the cervical spine. At this time, there is a growing body of literature critical of the evidence comparing arthroplasty with arthrodesis with respect to ASD incidence postoperatively. Points of contention regarding this topic include lack of long-term evidence, treatment group size disparities, as well as parameters used for evaluating ASD incidence within the study.

Nunley and colleagues[59] evaluated 173 patients among the FDA IDE trials for 4 different cervical disc replacement devices at 3 collaborating institutions with the primary aim of predicting the true incidence of symptomatic ASD after TDA in the cervical spine at 1 or 2 levels with median follow-up period of 4 years. The study concluded that the incidence of symptomatic ASD following cervical TDA is 3.1% annually regardless of the patient's sex, age, smoking habits, and design of disc prosthesis. They also noted that the presence of lumbar degenerative disease and osteopenia significantly increased the risk of developing ASD following anterior cervical surgery. Patients from the control group who underwent arthrodesis experienced an incidence of ASD at 2.8% annually. This difference between TDA and arthrodesis ASD annual incidence rate was not statistically significant.

Yin and colleagues[60] performed a meta-analysis of 10 randomized control trials involving 2227 patients, assessing functional scores, rates of reoperation, and major complications. Of the 10 trials, 6 trials, including 5 prospective, multicenter, FDA-regulated studies, were industry sponsored. The mean follow-up period of the 10 trials ranged from 1 to 5 years. Compared with ACDF, arthroplasty had better mean NDI, neurologic status, and a reduced incidence of reoperation related to the index surgery and major surgical complications. However, cervical disc arthroplasty did not reduce the risk of ASD any more than fusion. There was not a statistically significant difference between arthroplasty and arthrodesis in reoperation rates of adjacent segment levels at 4 to 5 years' average follow-up.

Another meta-analysis that sought to compare the reported incidence of ASD requiring surgical intervention between ACDF and TDA was performed by Verma and colleagues.[61] They obtained data from 6 prospective studies, including non-IDE and IDE trials with at least 2 years of follow-up with an overall sample size of 1586 patients (ACDF = 777, TDA = 809) with a final follow-up of 1110, giving an overall follow-up of 70%. At the conclusion of their study, they noted no difference in the rate of ASD for ACDF versus TDA.

Further investigation via prospective independent, randomized, blinded studies with long-term follow-up are necessary in order to assess the effects of arthroplasty compared with arthrodesis with respect to adjacent spinal segments. It has been evident from the literature that preexisting osteopenia and lumbar degenerative disc disease are contributing risk factors that significantly increase risk of ASD. Further assertions regarding the potential benefit of motion-sparing TDA compared with arthrodesis regarding ASD require further investigation and literature.

SUMMARY

Cervical TDA is a safe and effective surgical alternative to arthrodesis in patients with cervical radiculopathy or myelopathy. TDA helps obviate some of the complications associated with arthrodesis, such as graft site morbidity, allograft complications, and pseudarthrosis. Cervical TDA is also purported to have biomechanical advantages that may decrease the incidence of ASD compared with ACDF. Further long-term clinical data are necessary regarding the motion-sparing benefit with regard to ASD prevention in the TDA population compared with arthrodesis.

DISCLOSURE

K.E. Radcliff reports the following disclosures: 4 Web Medical, stock or stock options; 4Web, paid consultant; AAOS, board or committee member; Aesculap/B. Braun, research support; Bioventus, other financial or material support; Cervical Spine Research Society, board or committee member; DePuy, A Johnson & Johnson Company, other financial or material support; Globus Medical, intellectual property royalties; Innovative Spine Devices, intellectual property royalties; ISASS, board or committee member; North American Spine Society, board or committee member; Nuvasive, other financial or material support; Orthofix, Inc., research support; Rothman Institute, stock or stock options; Simplify Medical, research support; SMISS, board or committee member; Stryker, paid consultant; Synaptive Surgical, other financial or material support; Zimmer, unpaid consultant. G. Callanan reports no disclosures.

REFERENCES

1. Bohlman HH, Emery SE, Goodfellow DB, et al. Robinson anterior cervical discectomy and arthrodesis for cervical radiculopathy. Long-term follow-up of one hundred and twenty-two patients. J Bone Joint Surg 1993;75A:1298–307.
2. Goffin J, Geusens E, Vantomme N, et al. Long-term follow-up after interbody fusion of the cervical spine. J Spinal Disord Tech 2004;17:79–85.
3. Wang JC, McDonough PW, Endow KK, et al. Increased fusion rates with cervical plating for two-level anterior cervical discectomy and fusion. Spine 2000;25:41–5.
4. Hilibrand AS, Carlson GD, Palumbo MA, et al. Radiculopathy and myelopathy at segments adjacent to the site of a previous anterior cervical arthrodesis. J Bone Joint Surg 1999;81A:519–28.
5. Mutoh N, Shinomiya K, Furuya K, et al. Pseudarthrosis and delayed union after anterior cervical fusion. Int Orthop 1993;17:286–9.
6. Simmons EH. Anterior cervical discectomy and fusion. Proc R Soc Med 1970;63:897–8.
7. Kannan A, HSU WK, Sasso RC. Cervical disc replacement. Rothman-Simeone and Herkowitz's the Spine. Philadelphia, PA: Elsevier; 2018. p. 771–84.
8. Robertson PA, Wray AC. Natural history of posterior iliac crest bone graft donation for spinal surgery: a prospective analysis of morbidity. Spine 2001;26: 1473–6.
9. Behairy YM, Al-Sebai W. A modified technique for harvesting full-thickness iliac crest bone graft. Spine 2001;26:695–7.
10. Hsu EL, Ghodasra JH, Ashtekar A, et al. A comparative evaluation of factors influencing osteoinductivity among scaffolds designed for bone regeneration. Tissue Eng A 2013;19:1764–72.
11. Hsu WK, Polavarapu M, Riaz R, et al. Nanocomposite therapy as a more efficacious and less inflammatory alternative to bone morphogenetic protein-2 in a rodent arthrodesis model. J Orthop Res 2011; 29:1812–9.
12. Cummins BH, Robertson JT, Gill SS. Surgical experience with an implanted artificial cervical joint. J Neurosurg 1998;88:943–8.
13. Mummaneni PV, Haid RW. The future in the care of the cervical spine: interbody fusion and arthroplasty. Invited submission from the Joint Section Meeting on Disorders of the Spine and Peripheral Nerves, March 2004. J Neurosurg Spine 2004;1: 155–9.
14. Galbusera F, Bellini CM, Brayda-Bruno M, et al. Biomechanical studies on cervical total disc

arthroplasty: a literature review. Clin Biomech (Bristol, Avon) 2008;23:1095–104.

15. DiAngelo DJ, Foley KT, Morrow BR, et al. In vitro biomechanics of cervical disc arthroplasty with the ProDisc-C total disc implant. Neurosurg Focus 2004;17:E7.

16. Puttlitz CM, Rousseau MA, Xu Z, et al. Intervertebral disc replacement maintains cervical spine kinetics. Spine 2004;29:2809–14.

17. Rabin D, Pickett GE, Bisnaire L, et al. The kinematics of anterior cervical discectomy and fusion versus artificial cervical disc: a pilot study. Neurosurgery 2007;61:100–4.

18. Sasso RC, Best NM, Metcalf NH, et al. Motion analysis of bryan cervical disc arthroplasty versus anterior discectomy and fusion: results from a prospective, randomized, multicenter, clinical trial. J Spinal Disord Tech 2008;21:393–9.

19. Gandhi AA, Kode S, DeVries NA, et al. Biomechanical analysis of cervical disc replacement and fusion using single level, two level and hybrid constructs. Spine 2015;40(20):1578–85.

20. Mummaneni PV, Burkus JK, Haid RW, et al. Clinical and radiographic analysis of cervical disc arthroplasty compared with allograft fusion: a randomized controlled clinical trial. J Neurosurg Spine 2007;6:198–209.

21. Riew KD, Buchowski JM, Sasso R, et al. Cervical disc arthroplasty compared with arthrodesis for the treatment of myelopathy. J Bone Joint Surg Am 2008;90A:2354–64.

22. Kasliwal MK, Traynelis VC. "Cervical total disc arthroplasty." Benzel's Spine Surgery. Philadelphia, PA: Saunders; 2016. p. 1587–90.

23. Campbell PG, Yadla S, Malone J, et al. Early complications related to approach in cervical spine surgery: single-center prospective study. World Neurosurg 2010;74:363–8.

24. Riley LH 3rd, Skolasky RL, Albert TJ, et al. Dysphagia after anterior cervical decompression and fusion: prevalence and risk factors from a longitudinal cohort study. Spine 2005;30:2564–9.

25. Kasliwal MK, Traynelis VC. Motion preservation in cervical spine: review. J Neurosurg Sci 2012;56:13–25.

26. Mummaneni PV, Robinson JC, Haid RW Jr. Cervical arthroplasty with the Prestige LP cervical disc. Neurosurgery 2007;60:310–4 [discussion: 314–5].

27. Pickett GE, Mitsis DK, Sekhon LH, et al. Effects of a cervical disc prosthesis on segmental and cervical spine alignment. Neurosurg Focus 2004;17:E5.

28. van Loon J, Goffin J. Unanticipated outcomes after cervical disk arthroplasty. Semin Spine Surg 2012;24:20–4.

29. Walraevens J, Demaerel P, Suetens P, et al. Longitudinal prospective long-term radiographic follow-up after treatment of single-level cervical disk disease with the Bryan Cervical. Disc Neurosurg 2010;67:679–87.

30. Bentley G, Dowd GS. Surgical treatment of arthritis in the elderly. Clin Rheum Dis 1986;12:291–327.

31. Cavanaugh DA, Nunley PD, Kerr EJ 3rd, et al. Delayed hyper- reactivity to metal ions after cervical disc arthroplasty: a case report and literature review. Spine 2009;34:E262–5.

32. Shim CS, Shin HD, Lee SH. Posterior avulsion fracture at adjacent vertebral body during cervical disc replacement with ProDisc-C: a case report. J Spinal Disord Tech 2007;20:468–72.

33. Burkus JK, Haid RW, Traynelis VC, et al. Long-term clinical and radiographic outcomes of cervical disc replacement with the Prestige disc: results from a prospective randomized controlled clinical trial. J Neurosurg Spine 2010;13:308–18.

34. Gornet MF, Burkus JK, Shaffrey ME, et al. Cervical disc arthroplasty with PRESTIGE LP disc versus anterior cervical discectomy and fusion: a prospective, multicenter investigational device exemption study. J Neurosurg Spine 2015;23(5):558–73.

35. Gornet MF, Lanman TH, Burkus JK, et al. Two-level cervical disc arthroplasty versus anterior cervical discectomy and fusion: 10-year outcomes of a prospective, randomized investigational device exemption clinical trial. J Neurosurg Spine 2019;1–11. https://doi.org/10.3171/2019.4.SPINE19157.

36. Sasso R, Martin L. The Bryan artificial disc. In: Yue J, editor. Motion preservation surgery of the spine: advanced techniques and controversies. Philadelphia: Saunders/Elsevier; 2008. p. 193–4.

37. Heller JG, Sasso RC, Papadopoulos SM, et al. Comparison of BRYAN cervical disc arthroplasty with anterior cervical decompression and fusion: clinical and radiographic results of a randomized, controlled, clinical trial. Spine 2009;34:101–7.

38. Sasso RC, Anderson PA, Riew KD, et al. Results of cervical arthroplasty compared with anterior discectomy and fusion: four-year clinical outcomes in a prospective, randomized controlled trial. J Bone Joint Surg 2011;93A:1684–92.

39. Zhao Y, Zhang Y, Sun Y, et al. Application of cervical arthroplasty with Bryan cervical disc: 10-year follow-up results in China. Spine (Phila Pa 1976) 2016;41(2):111–5.

40. Delamarter R, Pradhan B. ProDisc-C total cervical disc replacement. In: Yue J, editor. Motion preservation surgery of the spine: advanced techniques and controversies. Philadelphia: Saunders/Elsevier; 2008. p. 214–5.

41. Murrey D, Janssen M, Delamarter R, et al. Results of the prospective, randomized, controlled multicenter Food and Drug Administration investigational device exemption study of the ProDisc-C total disc replacement versus anterior discectomy and fusion for the

treatment of 1-level symptomatic cervical disc disease. Spine J 2009;9(4):275–86.

42. Zigler JE, Delamarter R, Murrey D, et al. ProDisc-C and anterior cervical discectomy and fusion as surgical treatment for single-level cervical symptomatic degenerative disc disease: five-year results of a Food and Drug Administration study. Spine 2013; 38:203–9.

43. Kelly MP, Mok JM, Frisch RF, et al. Adjacent segment motion after anterior cervical discectomy and fusion versus Prodisc-C cervical total disk arthroplasty: analysis from a randomized, controlled trial. Spine 2011;36:1171–9.

44. Gornet MF, Burkus JK, Shaffrey ME, et al. Cervical disc arthroplasty with prestige LP disc versus anterior cervical discectomy and fusion: seven-year outcomes. Int J Spine Surg 2016;10:24.

45. Kim SH, Shin HC, Shin DA, et al. Early clinical experience with the Mobi-C disc prosthesis. Yonsei Med J 2007;48:457–64.

46. Park JH, Roh KH, Cho JY, et al. Comparative analysis of cervical arthroplasty using Mobi-C and anterior cervical discectomy and fusion using the Solis Cage. J Korean Neurosurg Soc 2008;44:217–21.

47. Guerin P, Obeid I, Gille O, et al. Sagittal alignment after single cervical disc arthroplasty. J Spinal Disord Tech 2012;25:10–6.

48. Beaurain J, Bernard P, Dufour T, et al. Intermediate clinical and radiological results of cervical TDR (Mobi-C) with up to 2 years of follow-up. Eur Spine J 2009;18:841–50.

49. Davis RJ, Kim KD, Hisey MS, et al. Cervical total disc replacement with the Mobi-C cervical artificial disc compared with anterior discectomy and fusion for treatment of 2-level symptomatic degenerative disc disease: a prospective, randomized, controlled multicenter clinical trial. J Neurosurg Spine 2013; 19:532–45.

50. Radcliff K, Davis RJ, Hisey MS, et al. "Long-term evaluation of cervical disc arthroplasty with the Mobi-C© cervical disc: a randomized, prospective, multicenter clinical trial with seven-year follow-up". Int J Spine Surg 2017;11(4):31.

51. Li J, Liang L, Ye XF, et al. Cervical arthroplasty with discover prosthesis: clinical outcomes and analysis of factors that may influence postoperative range of motion. Eur Spine J 2013;22(10):2303–9.

52. Skeppholm M, Lindgren L, Henriques T, et al. The discover artificial disc replacement versus fusion in cervical radiculopathy—a randomized controlled outcome trial with 2-year follow-up. Spine J 2015; 15(6):1284–94.

53. Stieber J, Fischgrund J, Abitbol J. The cervicore cervical intervertebral disc replacement. In: Yue J, editor. Motion preservation surgery of the spine: advanced techniques and controversies. Philadelphia: Saunders/Elsevier; 2008. p. 238–41.

54. Colle KO, Butler JB, Reyes PM, et al. Biomechanical evaluation of a metal-on-metal cervical intervertebral disc prosthesis. Spine J 2013;13(11):1640–9.

55. Rushton S, Marzluff J, McConnel J. SECURE-C cervical artificial disc. In: Yue J, editor. Motion preservation surgery of the spine: advanced techniques and controversies. Philadelphia: Saunders/Elsevier; 2008. p. 247–53.

56. Vaccaro A, Beutler W, Peppelman W, et al. Clinical outcomes with selectively constrained SECURE-C cervical disc arthroplasty: two-year results from a prospective, randomized, controlled, multi- center investigational device exemption study. Spine (Phila Pa 1976) 2013;38(26):2227–39.

57. Reyes-Sanchez A, Patwardhan A, Block J. The M6 artificial cervical disc. In: Yue J, editor. Motion preservation surgery of the spine: advanced techniques and controversies. Philadelphia: Saunders/Elsevier; 2008. p. 272–6.

58. Reyes-Sanchez A, Miramontes V, Olivarez LM, et al. Initial clinical experience with a next-generation artificial disc for the treatment of symptomatic degenerative cervical radiculopathy. SAS J 2010;4(1):9–15.

59. Nunley PD, Jawahar A, Cavanaugh DA, et al. Symptomatic adjacent segment disease after cervical total disc replacement: re-examining the clinical and radiological evidence with established criteria. Spine J 2013;13:5–12.

60. Yin S, Yu X, Zhou S, et al. Is cervical disc arthroplasty superior to fusion for treatment of symptomatic cervical disc disease? A meta-analysis. Clin Orthop Relat Res 2013;471:1904–19.

61. Verma K, Gandhi SD, Maltenfort M, et al. Rate of adjacent segment disease in cervical disc arthroplasty versus single-level fusion: meta-analysis of prospective studies. Spine 2013;38:2253–7.

Cervical Total Disc Replacement
Complications and Complication Avoidance

Richard L. Price, MD, PhD[a,b], Domagoj Coric, MD[c], Wilson Z. Ray, MD[a,*]

KEYWORDS

• Heterotopic ossification • Osteolysis • Complications • Subsidence • Focal device kyphosis

KEY POINTS

• Cervical total disc replacement (CTDR) has a unique set of complications compared to anterior cervical discectomy and fusion (ACDF). Proper patient selection and astute surgical technique can minimize the complication rate.
• As seen in other joint replacement procedures, heterotopic ossification (HO) and osteolysis are common in CTDR. Most of the time it is not symptomatic and only needs to be observed.
• Revision should be considered for complications that cause symptomatology. Oftentimes, revision motion-sparing procedures (ie, revision CTDR or posterior foraminotomy) can be performed, however, revision fusion may be the best option in some cases.

INTRODUCTION

CTDR is a motion-preserving operation for cervical spondylosis. Current indications include myelopathy or radiculopathy resulting from degenerative disc disease. In recent years it has emerged as an alternative to the gold standard treatment of anterior cervical discectomy and fusion (ACDF).[1] With careful patient selection and meticulous surgical technique, arthroplasty is an excellent motion preservation option.[2,3] With new any new technology come new types of complications, which can be generalized into short-term versus mid- and long-term complications. There are conflicting results comparing short-term complication rates between CTDR and ACDF, with most industry-sponsored trials showing a lower complication rate for CTDR, some authors have suggested that conflicts of interest may exist in industry-sponsored trials.[4] A recent large series of 52,395 patients by Kelly and colleagues.[5] showed similar short-term complication rates between CDTR

and ACDF when adjusted for pr-operative comorbidities.[5]

Short-term complication rates (**Table 1**) [less than 30 days] are thought to be related to the surgical approach. As CDTR and ACDF have the same anterior cervical surgical approach, it is intuitive that the complication rate is similar. These complications include dysphagia, infection, dural tear, major vessel injury, Horner syndrome, and recurrent laryngeal nerve injury. Dysphagia is the most common complication in both procedures. Depending on the series, the dysphagia complication rate in CTDR can range from 2% to 67%. The rates of dysphagia are highest in the immediate postoperative period.[6] Dysphagia is so common postoperatively that some surgeons suggest that it is an unavoidable outcome of anterior cervical surgery.[7] Some studies show no difference in dysphagia between CTDR and ACDF.[8] Meanwhile, several other meta-analyses suggest a lower rate of dysphagia in patients undergoing CTDR as compared to ACDF.[9,10] This

[a] Department of Neurological Surgery, Washington University School of Medicine, Campus Box 8057, 660 South Euclid Avenue, St Louis, MO 63110, USA; [b] Swedish Neuroscience Institute, Seattle, WA, USA; [c] Carolinas Neurosurgical and Spine Associates, 225 Baldwin Avenue, Charlotte, NC 28204, USA
* Corresponding author.
E-mail address: RayZ@wustl.edu

Neurosurg Clin N Am 32 (2021) 473–481
https://doi.org/10.1016/j.nec.2021.05.006
1042-3680/21/

Table 1
Complications

Short-Term Complications (Similar to ACDF)	Mid- to Long-Term Complications (Unique to CTDR)
Infection	Metallosis/immune reaction
Major vessel injury	Osteolysis
Horner syndrome	Heterotopic ossification
Recurrent laryngeal nerve injury	Focal device kyphosis
Esophageal injury	Subsidence
Dysphagia[a]	Vertebral body fracture
	Displacement
	Expulsion

Short-term complications for CTDR are similar to ACDF. Mid- to long-term complications of CTDR are unique.
[a] Potentially lower rate in CTDR.

phenomenon is believed to be caused by less anterior prominence of arthroplasty devices, which causes less irritation on the oropharynx, leading to a lower rate of dysphagia in the short-term postoperative period.[11]

After the early postoperative period, the types of complications for CTDR compared to ACDF diverge. CTDR patients experience a unique set of complications in the mid- to long-term time period. This chapter will critically examine complications unique to the CTDR procedure. Complications can generally be characterized as either an error in patient selection or surgical technique.[12] Patient selection is critical for CTDR success. Patients with osteoporosis, sagittal plane deformities, segmental pathologic motion, or advanced spondylitic disease are not good candidates for CTDR. When performing CTDR, the surgical technique is critical to success. There are many pitfalls that can lead to surgical failure and the need for reoperation. This chapter will focus on complications specific to CTDR as well as tips to avoid CTDR complications.

Device-Related Complications

In rare instances, surgical failure can be attributed solely to the surgical device. Reporting for these types of rare complications is mostly in the form of case reports. Device-related complications are either related to an immune reaction to the device or mechanical malfunction of the device. As in large joint arthroplasty, metallosis can occur with cervical arthroplasty devices.[13] Metallosis is an uncommon complication in arthroplasty. It is a result of metal debris from the implant infiltrating soft tissue adjacent to the implant. Metallosis in CTDR typically is not an issue. However, in rare cases metal debris may lead to reactive tissue that can cause compression of neural elements, in which case surgical decompression is warranted. Additionally, immune responses to the implant have been documented.[14] In these cases there is a histopathologic lymphocytic reaction to the implant, resulting in a local mass effect that creates symptomatology. Both metallosis and immune reaction to the implant are underreported since most cases are asymptomatic. Experience with cervical arthroplasty devices have proven their durability thus far. Reports of device fracture are rare, in both reports the fracture occurred in the ceramic portion of the device[15,16] At this point in time only rare case reports have demonstrated cervical arthroplasty device failure. There are certainly other cases that have not been reported in the literature. Also, with extended follow-up of patients additional failures will certainly be encountered. In all cases of device failure, reoperation with conversion to ACDF was the treatment modality of choice.

Heterotopic Ossification

Heterotopic ossification (HO) is a phenomenon well-published in orthopedic joint replacement literature. HO is defined as bone formation outside of the skeletal system. In CTDR patients, HO occurs around the implant, and was first reported in 2005.[17] Excessive bone formation can lead to bridging ossification, which in turn effectively fuses the spinal segment (**Figs. 1–3**). The resultant fusion defeats the purpose of placing a motion-sparing device. The HO rates following CTDR vary wildly. Different published series range from a rate of 7.3% to 69.2%.[18–21] The highly variable nature of HO may be confounded by how the degree of HO is quantified and also variability in follow-up within different studies. To better quantify the extent of HO, Mehren and colleagues developed a classification system for HO[20] (**Table 2**). The scale ranges from 0 (no HO) to IV (complete fusion with no movement on flexion/extension x-rays). The grading system is useful to objectively determine the extent of HO in follow-up and how it affects cervical spine mobility. A pooled average between multiple studies suggests HO occurs in 44.6% of patients. In a long-term study, 53% of patients had some evidence of HO at 5 years and beyond.[21] Additionally, large meta-analyses show that the rate of HO increases with time, suggesting that HO is a dynamic process that can manifest late in the postoperative course.[22] Yi

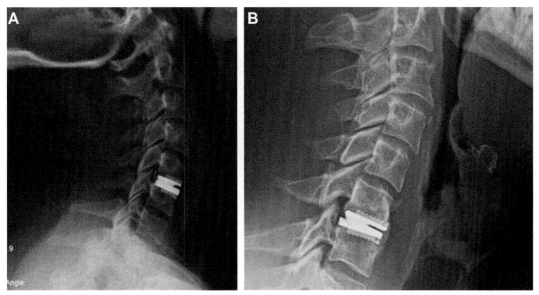

Fig. 1. Lateral cervical x-ray demonstrating heterotopic ossification (*A*) posterior and (*B*) anterior to implant.

and colleagues demonstrated that older age and male sex are risk factors for HO development.[23] Despite a high rate of occurrence, HO rarely causes symptoms and typically does not need revision surgery. Unfortunately, severe and progressive HO may lead to bridging ossification that fuses the index level, which defeats the purpose of using a motion-sparing device over ACDF.

Several strategies exist to reduce HO formation intraoperatively. Exposed cancellous bone promotes HO, so care should be taken to minimize unroofing cancellous bone with generous waxing of bleeding bone. Excessive drilling of the endplates should be avoided. When drilling, copious irrigation is recommended. Although HO is a dynamic process that occurs over time it is felt that the majority of HO occurs within the first 100 days postoperatively. During this time, supplementation with NSAIDs is recommended to help prevent HO. The authors recommend ibuprofen 600 mg TID for 6 weeks after surgery.

Osteolysis

Osteolysis is described as the vertebral body bone loss at the index level after a CTDR procedure. Bone loss is typically found on the anterior edge of the superior vertebral body of the index level. Some degree of osteolysis after CTDR is common, occurring in more than 50% of cases.[24] Despite a high prevalence of occurrence of osteolysis, it is rarely symptomatic and typically does not require revision surgery.[25] Heo and colleagues developed a grading system for bone loss following arthroplasty. In their series, 60.4% of patients experienced some degree of osteolysis with 8/48 (16.7%) experiencing grade 3 osteolysis, defined as the anterior portion of the disc being exposed due to bone loss. Despite extensive loss of bone, no patients underwent revision surgery.[26] Interestingly, osteolysis typically occurs within the first postoperative year, but rarely progresses after 1-year.[24,26,27] With continued bone erosion, additional failure such as device subsidence and segmental kyphosis can occur. In these instances,

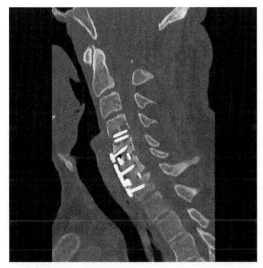

Fig. 2. Sagittal CT demonstrating osteolysis adjacent to the arthroplasty implant at C4 and C5.

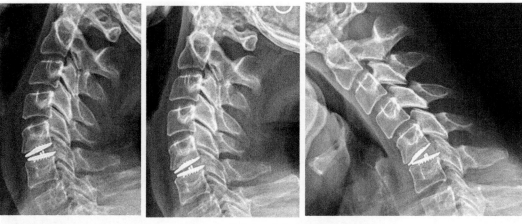

Fig. 3. Flexion/extension cervical x-ray demonstrating focal device kyphosis C5/6.

surgical correction is often necessary if the patient is symptomatic. If encountered, we recommend close radiological follow-up until bone loss has stabilized as defined by imaging.

Bone loss following large joint arthroplasty is a well-documented phenomenon. Though the mechanisms of bone loss are not entirely understood, some mechanisms that have been suggested in large joint bone loss include foreign body reaction of the implant, wear debris effect, micromotion at the bone/prothesis interface, and stress-shielding effects.[28–31] All of these mechanisms may play a part in bone loss in CTDR. Whenever there is progressive bone loss, indolent infection should be ruled out as a cause of osteolysis. *Cutibacterium acnes* is a notorious offender in device-related infections. If suspected, multiple specimens should be obtained and cultures allowed to grow for at least 10 days to reduce diagnostic error.[32] Thermal injury from electrocautery is hypothesized as another mechanism for bone loss encountered in CTDR. The heat generated may initiate a cascade of osteoclastic gene expression and destruction of vasculature leading to depletion of bone.[27,33,34] Another proposed mechanism of bone loss is the loading force of the implant that is distributed on the posterior aspect of the vertebral body. Along these lines, implants with large shell angles were associated with more severe bone loss.[27] Osteolysis is seen with all FDA-approved devices, yet one study suggests that the Mobi-C device has the highest rate of osteolysis.[24]

Subsidence

Subsidence is defined as sinking of the implant into vertebral endplates. This results in disc space collapse with associated foraminal stenosis. Clinically, this can present as axial neck pain or radiculopathy. Subsidence of the implant may lead to a reduction of movement through the index level. This can overload adjacent levels leading to adjacent segment disease. Implant subsidence has been reported in up to one-third of cases and has been reported up to 4 years postoperatively.[35] However, clinically significant subsidence is less than 3% in large series.[36–38] Osteoporosis, osteopenia, and bone metabolic disorders increase the risk of subsidence. CTDR should be avoided in these patients.

Like HO, one mechanism of subsidence is endplate violation. Endplates must be carefully prepared to remove all disc, but not overdrilled as to avoid endplate violation. Subsidence is also

Table 2	
Mehren classification of heterotopic ossification	
Grade	**Characteristics of HO Grades**
0	No HO present
I	HO present in front of vertebral body, not in intradiscal space
II	HO present in intradiscal space, possible effect on implant function
III	Bridging HO, but movement of implant
IV	Complete fusion with no movement with flexion/extension

McAfee PC, Cunningham BW, Devine J, et al. Classification of heterotopic ossification (HO) in artificial disk replacement. J Spinal Disord Tech 2003;16:384-9.

commonly associated with implant under- or over-sizing. Biomechanical data show that undersized implants increase stress concentrations per unit area of the endplate, which in turn increases the risk of implant subsidence.[39] When selecting appropriate implant intraoperatively, careful attention should be paid to make sure the implant covers as much of the endplate as possible to minimize subsidence risk.

Vertebral Body Fracture

Vertebral body fractures after CTDR are rare. Most fractures are correlated with implant design or poor surgical technique. Also, there have been rare reports of vertebral body fractures in CTDR patients after trauma.[40] Fractures are more commonly seen in multilevel CTDRs, particularly when using implants with a keel. Any cervical arthroplasty implant may cause a vertebral body fracture, but are most common with Pro-disc implants because of the large keel.[41] When performing multilevel CTDR, we recommend choosing implants with a small keel. Also, meticulous care needs to be taken to avoid placing implant keels vertically in line with each other, as this can lead to a sagittal split fracture.[42] Poor surgical technique can also lead to a vertebral body fracture. Shallow keel cuts can result in fracture propagation that extends throughout the vertebral body when placing the implant.

Vertebral body fractures may clinically present as axial neck pain. Fractures that propagate may lead to implant loosening. As implants loosen, they can subside, lead to focal device kyphosis, or even device migration. Oftentimes, vertebral body fractures become symptomatic and require a larger revision surgery, such as a corpectomy, to stabilize the fracture. If a fracture is suspected, CT imaging is critical to objectively define the extent of the fracture and to determine if surgical correction is necessary or if close radiological observation is sufficient.

SUBOPTIMAL DEVICE PLACEMENT

Precise device sizing is paramount for CTDR replacement. Under- or oversizing an implant can lead to several disastrous complications. Unlike other CTDR complications, such as HO or osteolysis, suboptimal device placement often needs surgical correction. Focal device kyphosis was first reported in 2004.[43] In their study utilizing the Bryan artificial disc, Johnson and colleagues, showed a focal loss of lordosis of about 4° at the index level. This focal loss of lordosis did not affect the overall cervical lordosis of the patient. Interestingly, patients with two-level CTDR did not see any change in focal lordosis. One mechanism proposed is overmilling the endplates, specifically the anterior portion. As in other types of CTDR complications, it is critical to not overdrill vertebral endplates as this can cause a suboptimal surface for the dynamic implant to integrate.

Rare, but disastrous, types of suboptimal device placement are displacement and expulsion. Displacement of implant is when a portion, typically a footplate, becomes dislodged (**Fig. 4**A). The dislodged portion can migrate anteriorly and irritate the retropharyngeal space. Theoretically, a portion of the implant could become displaced posteriorly, but to the authors' knowledge this has not been reported in the literature. Expulsion is ejection of the entire implant out of the disc space anteriorly (**Fig. 4**B). Both displacement and expulsion typically present with axial neck pain. Both complications must be revised surgically before the extruded implant can cause damage to surrounding tissue (ie, esophageal perforation). Both complications are most commonly caused by oversizing the implant in regards to disc height. It is critical for the surgeon not to become overzealous with implant sizing. Whereas it is common for an ACDF to use an 8- or 9-mm implant, CTDR typically should only require 5- or 6-mm implants, with rare placement of 7-mm implants. This smaller size is crucial to maintaining physiologic motion and avoid distraction of the facets. Maintaining neutral cervical spine positions helps to avoid postoperative device kyphosis.

Additionally, the authors suggest not placing the patient's head in traction when performing a CTDR. Even a small amount of distraction will artificially expand the disc height and lead to oversizing the implant. It is important to keep the patient's neck as physiologic as possible, in order to select the best implant that will be best suited to preserve motion in the patient. Excellent intraoperative fluoroscopy is critical to success for implant sizing. Perfect AP/lateral x-rays need to be obtained with the trial implant to best gauge how the implant will fit postoperatively. Many errors in implant sizing errors that will ultimately lead to focal segmental kyphosis, displacement, and expulsion can be identified and corrected intraoperatively.

Complication Mitigation and Surgical Revision

As stated earlier in this chapter, wise patient selection and excellent operative technique are the two biggest factors to reduce postoperative complications. Strictly adhering to patient selection criteria and resisting the urge to perform CTDR on

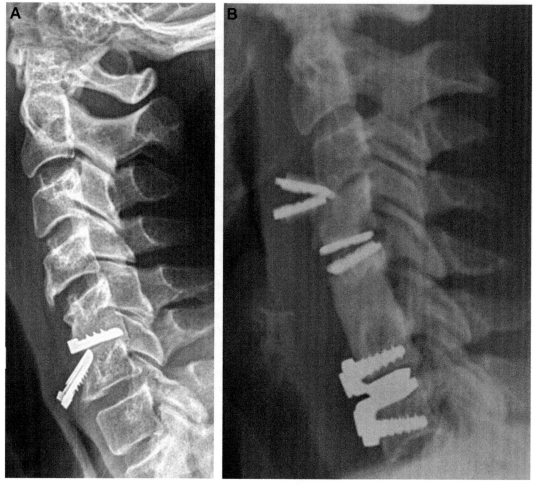

Fig. 4. Lateral x-ray showing device displacement (*A*) and expulsion (*B*).

nonideal candidates that opt for arthroplasty as opposed to fusion is the foundation to success. Intraoperatively, there are several techniques to mitigate CTDR-specific complications. The surgical goal of CTDR is to remove pathologic tissue to decompress neural elements and then insert a device that maintains natural movement. Minimizing damage to surrounding tissue is paramount. Electrocautery use has been associated with osteolysis. Bone wax should be used instead if possible, especially over exposed cancellous bone. Excessive drilling should be avoided also. Copious irrigation and avoiding drilling into endplates help reduces HO. Sizing of the implant must be meticulously evaluated with trial sizes before placing the actual implant. The implant should fill the disc space, but not overdistract the facets. A true AP radiograph should be acquired before making keel cuts to verify that the implant is midline. Ensuring ideal implant size will enable

physiologic motion, ultimately reducing mid- and long-term complications.

Many postoperative complications such as HO that are related to CTDR can be managed nonoperatively. After complications are recognized, close follow-up with imaging must occur. Development of symptoms or instability of the implant are indications for surgery. Skovrlj and colleagues evaluated 1068 CTDR levels with an average follow-up of 2.3 years. They determined the mean rate of reoperation, a surgery that does not alter the initial implant (ie, laminoforaminotomy) rate of about of 1.0%, revision rate of 0.2%, and 1.2% rate of removal and conversion to fusion.[44] Patients that present with recurrent radiculopathy at the index level often can undergo laminoforaminotomy for symptom relief. Minor subsidence can be managed with close follow-up. Persistent symptomatology warrants revision however. Minor subsidence with symptoms may be amenable to revision CTDR, but there should be a low threshold to convert to fusion. Corpectomy may be necessary for patients with major subsidence. Cases of symptomatic osteolysis should be converted to a fusion. If there is considerable bone loss, then a corpectomy is indicated. Expulsion or displacement of the device is typically converted to a fusion. Severe, multilevel revision may require posterior fusion as well as to restore alignment and stabilize the cervical spine.

Removal of the device can be challenging. The Synthes ProDisc-C and Medtronic Bryan disc have had removal guidelines published by the manufacturer.[45,46] For device removal, the patient should be placed in cervical traction during the case to assist in distracting the endplates. The implant can be accessed from the initial incision and then scar tissue and osteophytes must be removed from the implant–vertebral body interface. Once exposed, an osteotome can be used to separate the device from the vertebral body endplates. After adequate separation has been achieved, we recommend using a Kocher to gently pull the implant out of the disc space. It is usually easier to extract the components of the device instead of the entire device at once. After removal, carefully inspect all areas of the disc space for device debris before performing a salvage procedure. Explantation of the device should be reported to the manufacturer.

SUMMARY

CTDR has proven to be a durable, motion-sparing alternative to ACDF. However, there are unique complications associated with the procedure. Understanding the nature of these complications and how to mitigate risks will reduce undesired outcomes. Many complications, such as HO and osteolysis, can be carefully observed. Close follow-up is necessary with a low threshold to revise CTDR for new or persistent symptomatology. Careful patient selection and meticulous surgical technique help to mitigate the complication rate, ultimately making CTDR an appealing, motion-preserving option for treatment of cervical spondylitic disease. As there is a lack of late-term follow-up (>20 years), additional and unique complications associated with CTDR will surface. If able to extrapolate from large-joint arthroplasty, then there will be delayed device-related complications and failure. As time goes on, continued late-term follow-up and reporting of complications or device failures is necessary for the evolution and refinement of CTDR.

CLINICS CARE POINTS

- Patient selection and meticulous surgical technique are the cornerstone for reducing CTDR complications.
- Minimize drilling of endplates to avoid exposing cancellous bone.
- Copious amounts of bone wax should be applied to bleeding bone edges to reduce the HO rate.
- Perfect AP and lateral x-rays allow for ideal positioning of the implant.
- Avoid cervical traction for CTDR, proper implant sizing is critical to maintain normal flexion/extension motion.

DISCLOSURE

The authors have nothing to disclose.

REFERENCES

1. Kelly MP, Mok JM, Frisch RF, et al. Adjacent segment motion after anterior cervical discectomy and fusion versus prodisc-c cervical total disk arthroplasty. Spine 2011;36:1171–9.
2. Tortolani Pj, Moatz B. Cervical disc arthroplasty: pros and cons. Surg Neurol Int 2012;3:216.
3. Wenger M, Markwalder T-M. Bryan total disc arthroplasty: a replacement disc for cervical disc disease. Medi Devices (Auckl) 2010;3:11–24.
4. Ioannidis JPA. Adverse events in randomized trials: neglected, restricted, distorted, and silenced. Arch Intern Med 2009;169:1737–9.
5. Kelly MP, Eliasberg CD, Riley MS, et al. Reoperation and complications after anterior cervical discectomy and fusion and cervical disc arthroplasty: a study of 52,395 cases. Eur Spine J 2018;27:1432–9.
6. Rihn JA, Kane J, Albert TJ, et al. What is the incidence and severity of dysphagia after anterior cervical surgery? Clin Orthop Relat Res 2011;469:658–65.
7. Shriver MF, Lewis DJ, Kshettry VR, et al. Dysphagia rates after anterior cervical diskectomy and fusion: a systematic review and meta-analysis. Glob Spine J 2017;7:95–103.
8. Liu F-Y, Yang D-L, Huang W-Z, et al. Risk factors for dysphagia after anterior cervical spine surgery. Medicine 2017;96:e6267.
9. Zhong Z-M, Li M, Han Z-M, et al. Does cervical disc arthroplasty have lower incidence of dysphagia than

anterior cervical discectomy and fusion? A meta-analysis. Clin Neurol Neurosurg 2016;146:45–51.

10. Findlay C, Ayis S, Demetriades AK. Total disc replacement versus anterior cervical discectomy and fusion: a systematic review with meta-analysis of data from a total of 3160 patients across 14 randomized controlled trials with both short- and medium- to long-term outcomes. Bone Joint J 2018; 100-B:991–1001.

11. Skeppholm M, Olerud C. Comparison of dysphagia between cervical artificial disc replacement and fusion: data from a randomized controlled study with two years of follow-up. Spine 2013;38:E1507–10.

12. Parish JM, Asher AM, Coric D. Complications and complication avoidance with cervical total disc replacement. Int J Spine Surg 2020;14:S50–6.

13. Cavanaugh DA, Nunley PD, Kerr EJ, et al. Delayed hyper-reactivity to metal ions after cervical disc arthroplasty. Spine 2009;34:E262–5.

14. Guyer RD, Shellock J, MacLennan B, et al. Early failure of metal-on-metal artificial disc prostheses associated with lymphocytic reaction. Spine 2011;36: E492–7.

15. Nguyen NQ, Kafle D, Buchowski JM, et al. Ceramic fracture following cervical disc arthroplasty. J Bone Joint Surg Am 2011;93:e132.

16. Fan H, Wu S, Wu Z, et al. Implant failure of bryan cervical disc due to broken polyurethane sheath. Spine 2012;37:E814–6.

17. Parkinson JF, Sekhon LHS. Cervical arthroplasty complicated by delayed spontaneous fusion: case report. J Neurosurg Spine 2005;2:377–80.

18. Wu J-C, Huang W-C, Tsai H-W, et al. Differences between 1- and 2-level cervical arthroplasty: more heterotopic ossification in 2-level disc replacement: clinical article. J Neurosurg Spine 2012;16:594–600.

19. Yi S, Kim KN, Yang MS, et al. Difference in occurrence of heterotopic ossification according to prosthesis type in the cervical artificial disc replacement. Spine 2010;35:1556–61.

20. Mehren C, Suchomel P, Grochulla F, et al. Heterotopic ossification in total cervical artificial disc replacement. Spine 2006;31:2802–6.

21. Chen J, Wang X, Bai W, et al. Prevalence of heterotopic ossification after cervical total disc arthroplasty: a meta-analysis. Eur Spine J 2011;21: 674–80.

22. Kong L, Ma Q, Meng F, et al. The prevalence of heterotopic ossification among patients after cervical artificial disc replacement. Medicine 2017;96:e7163.

23. Leung C, Casey ATh, Goffin J, et al. Clinical significance of heterotopic ossification in cervical disc replacement: a prospective multicenter clinical trial. Neurosurgery 2005;57:759–63.

24. Kieser DC, Cawley DT, Fujishiro T, et al. Risk factors for anterior bone loss in cervical disc arthroplasty. J Neurosurg Spine 2018;29:123–9.

25. Joaquim AF, Lee NJ, Lehman RA, et al. Osteolysis after cervical disc arthroplasty. Eur Spine J 2020; 1–11.

26. Heo DH, Lee DC, Oh JY, et al. Bone loss of vertebral bodies at the operative segment after cervical arthroplasty: a potential complication? Neurosurg Focus 2017;42:E7.

27. Chen T-Y, Chen W-H, Tzeng C-Y, et al. Anterior bone loss after cervical Bryan disc arthroplasty: insight into the biomechanics following total disc replacement. Spine J 2020;20:1211–8.

28. Boyle C, Kim IY. Comparison of different hip prosthesis shapes considering micro-level bone remodeling and stress-shielding criteria using three-dimensional design space topology optimization. J Biomech 2011;44:1722–8.

29. Fraser J, Werner S, Jacofsky D. Wear and loosening in total knee arthroplasty: a quick review. J Knee Surg 2014;28:139–44.

30. Chen C-M, Tsai W-C, Lin S-C, et al. Effects of stemmed and nonstemmed hip replacement on stress distribution of proximal femur and implant. BMC Musculoskelet Disord 2014;15:312.

31. Gallo J, Goodman SB, Konttinen YT, et al. Osteolysis around total knee arthroplasty: a review of pathogenetic mechanisms. Acta Biomater 2013;9: 8046–58.

32. Hsu JE, Bumgarner RE, Matsen FA. Propionibacterium in shoulder arthroplasty: what we think we know today. J Bone Joint Surg Am 2016;98:597–606.

33. Dolan EB, Haugh MG, Voisin MC, et al. Thermally induced osteocyte damage initiates a remodelling signaling cascade. PLoS One 2015;10:e0119652.

34. Dolan EB, Tallon D, Cheung W-Y, et al. Thermally induced osteocyte damage initiates pro-osteoclastogenic gene expression in vivo. J R Soc Interf 2016;13:20160337.

35. Hacker FM, Babcock RM, Hacker RJ. Very late complications of cervical arthroplasty: results of 2 controlled randomized prospective studies from a single investigator site. Spine 2013;38:2223–6.

36. Vaccaro A, Beutler W, Peppelman W, et al. Long-term clinical experience with selectively constrained SECURE-C cervical artificial disc for 1-level cervical disc disease: results from seven-year follow-up of a prospective, randomized, controlled investigational device exemption clinical trial. Int J Spine Surg 2018;12:377–87.

37. Wang L, Hu B, Wang L, et al. Clinical and radiographic outcome of dynamic cervical implant (DCI) arthroplasty for degenerative cervical disc disease: a minimal five-year follow-up. BMC Musculoskelet Disord 2018;19:101.

38. Gornet MF, Burkus JK, Shaffrey ME, et al. Cervical disc arthroplasty with prestige LP disc versus anterior cervical discectomy and fusion: seven-year outcomes. Int J Spine Surg 2016;10:24.

39. Lin C-Y, Kang H, Rouleau JP, et al. Stress analysis of the interface between cervical vertebrae end plates and the Bryan, Prestige LP, and ProDisc-C cervical disc prostheses: an in vivo image-based finite element study. Spine 2009;34:1554–60.

40. Salari B, McAfee PC. Cervical total disk replacement: complications and avoidance. Orthop Clin North Am 2012;43:97–107.

41. Shim CS, Lee S, Maeng DH, et al. Vertical split fracture of the vertebral body following total disc replacement using ProDisc: report of two cases. J Spinal Disord Tech 2005;18:465–9.

42. Datta JC, Janssen ME, Beckham R, et al. Sagittal split fractures in multilevel cervical arthroplasty using a keeled prosthesis. J Spinal Disord Tech 2007;20:89–92.

43. Johnson JP, Lauryssen C, Cambron HO, et al. Sagittal alignment and the Bryan cervical artificial disc. Neurosurg Focus 2004;17:1–4.

44. Reoperations following cervical disc replacement. Asian Spine J 2015;1–12.

45. Spine S. ProDisc-C removal system: instruments to assist with the removal of the ProDisc-C total disc replacement device. Available at: http://sites.synthes.com/MediaBin/US%20DATA/Product%20Support%20Materials/Technique%20Guides/SPINE/SPTGProDisc-CRemovalJ10359A.pdf. Accessed November 20, 2020.

46. Medtronic, ACD instrument set: surgical technique shown with the Bryan cervical disc system. Available at: http://www.forma-cionencirugia.com/archivos/BRYAN%20ACD%20ST%20NUEVA.pdf. Accessed November 18, 2020.

Cervical Spine Surgery
Arthroplasty Versus Fusion Versus Posterior Foraminotomy

Vincent Rossi, MD, MBA[a,b,*], Tim Adamson, MD[a,b]

KEYWORDS

- ACDF • Arthroplasty • CTDR • Foraminotomy • Minimally invasive

KEY POINTS

- Three procedures predominate for surgical management of degenerative cervical spine disorders: posterior cervical laminoforaminotomy, cervical total disc replacement, and anterior cervical discectomy and fusion.
- The 3 procedures together provide a 360° approach to degenerative cervical spine disease that, when combined with patient preference, helps to reach the correct treatment decision.
- Additional considerations of minimally invasive technique, outpatient setting, motion preservation, and adjacent-segment disease should be taken into consideration when formulating a surgical plan.
- It should be the goal of all well-rounded spine surgeons to be skilled at both anterior and posterior approaches to treat radiculopathy, and then to select the most appropriate for the patient's individual disorder.

INTRODUCTION

Degenerative cervical spine disease can present with broad symptoms. Often, these symptoms include axial neck pain, radiculopathy, myelopathy, or a combination. Radiographic findings can include disc herniation, cervical stenosis, foraminal stenosis, and/or cervical spondylosis. Three procedures predominate for surgical management of degenerative cervical spine disorders: posterior cervical laminoforaminotomy (PCF), cervical total disc replacement (CTDR), and anterior cervical discectomy and fusion (ACDF). These procedures have all proved to be safe and effective in the treatment of degenerative cervical spine disease. The decision of which procedure to use is not necessarily consistent for each imaging finding, presentation, and patient population. The 3 procedures together provide a 360° approach to degenerative cervical spine disease that, when combined with patient preference, help clinicians reach the correct treatment decision. Although these 3 procedures have diverse applications, they overlap most in equipoise for the treatment of unilateral cervical radiculopathy. As a result, this article discusses these procedures in the context of unilateral cervical radiculopathy. Ultimately, these procedures might all be effective in alleviating the clinical symptoms, but the choice of procedure may have additional consequences for the patient, including recovery time, adjacent-segment disease, and motion preservation.

BACKGROUND

Cervical radiculopathy is a common medical condition affecting up to 2.5 million people in the United States each year.[1] Most of those resolve with nonsurgical therapy measures, such as physical therapy, chiropractic care, and epidural

[a] Carolina Neurosurgery and Spine Associates, Atrium Health Musculoskeletal Institute, 225 Baldwin Avenue, Charlotte, NC 28204, USA; [b] Atrium Health Musculoskeletal Institute, 1000 Blythe Boulevard, Charlotte, NC 28203, USA
* Corresponding author.
E-mail address: vrossi89@gmail.com
Twitter: @vincentrossimd (V.R.)

Neurosurg Clin N Am 32 (2021) 483–492
https://doi.org/10.1016/j.nec.2021.05.005
1042-3680/21/© 2021 Elsevier Inc. All rights reserved.

steroid injections, but approximately one-fourth require surgery for relief of their symptoms. Although it affects almost all ages, it is most common from 50 to 54 years of age (1 out of 500), when people are at their most productive socioeconomically. The goal of any surgical intervention should be to resolve persistent radiculopathy symptoms, allow a rapid return to full productive life, and minimize risk for immediate and long-term sequelae as much as possible.

HISTORY

The origins of surgery for cervical radiculopathy go back more than 80 years with the pioneering work of Stookey.[1] By the 1940s and 1950s, Frykholm[2] and Murphey and Simmons [3] had standardized the open posterior cervical laminoforaminotomy technique and were publishing excellent results, with more than 90% good outcomes with a low (1.5%) complication rate. Over the ensuing decades, this technique was improved and became the benchmark of low risk and good outcome for spine surgery. During this same time, it also became apparent that not all forms of cervical spine disorder were amenable to a posterior approach. The initial work of Cloward[4] followed by Robinson and Smith[5] popularized the anterior decompression and fusion technique. Not only was this technique useful for the treatment of cervical radiculopathy, it allowed successful treatment of myelopathy and spinal deformities. The anterior approach quickly became the preferred approach and, at many institutions, the only approach for cervical radiculopathy.

As experience with anterior decompression and fusion grew, it became apparent that there were also complications unique to the anterior exposure and consequences to the levels adjacent to the fusion.[6] In spite of continued good outcomes in large series of open posterior laminoforaminotomy[6,7] and the addition of microsurgical technique to further minimize the trauma of the surgery, the anterior approach remained more popular and most cervical spine surgery literature focused on better ways to increase fusion rates with the introduction of plating systems.

ANTERIOR CERVICAL DISCECTOMY AND FUSION VERSUS CERVICAL TOTAL DISC REPLACEMENT VERSUS POSTERIOR CERVICAL LAMINOFORAMINOTOMY
Anterior Cervical Discectomy And Fusion

ACDF has been the gold-standard treatment of cervical soft disc herniation and cervical spondylotic disease since it was first described by Robinson

and Smith[5] in 1955.[7] This procedure allows complete discectomy, disc height restoration, direct and indirect foraminal decompression, central decompression, and removal of herniated nucleus pulposus (HNP). In addition, fusion across the disc space enhanced by interbody graft and plating results in stabilization. Despite ACDF having satisfactory results in 90% to 95% of patients, more attention has been focused on alternative surgical options.[6] Long-term follow-up of cervical fusion patients and a more nuanced understanding of biomechanical stresses of fusion have led to a greater appreciation of the negative effects that fusion has on adjacent-segment disease. Symptomatic adjacent-segment disease leading to reoperation has been reported to occur at a rate of 0.7% per year following ACDF.[8]

Cervical Total Disc Replacement

CTDR was first described by Cummins[9] in 1991.[10] The indications for CTDR are radiculopathy with 1-level or 2-level cervical soft disc herniation caused by central or paracentral disc herniation. One of the goals of motion preservation in CTDR is to reduce the rate of adjacent-segment disease. Benefits of CTDR include discectomy, disc height restoration, near-physiologic motion preservation, indirect decompression, and removal of HNP. There is extensive literature analyzing the incidence of adjacent-segment disease after CTDR, and, with follow-up approaching 10 years, some studies suggest a reduced incidence with CTDR.[11–14]

Posterior Cervical Laminoforaminotomy

PCF was first popularized by Spurling, Scoville, and Frykholm in the 1950s.[15,16] The minimally invasive cervical microendoscopic laminoforaminotomy (MELF) technique was described by Adamson[17–20] in 2001.[21] These procedures allow decompression of the neural foramen and retrieval of foraminal and some paracentral soft disc herniations. This technique is motion preserving and allows for substantial foraminal decompression. The use of this procedure is limited to foraminal disease given the limitations of performing central decompression from the posterior approach.

INDICATIONS

Degenerative cervical spine disease should undergo attempted nonsurgical therapies when appropriate. Such therapies include over-the-counter pain medications, nonsteroidal antiinflammatory drugs, physical therapy, and injections when appropriate. If failure to obtain relief of symptoms occurs, surgical intervention may be appropriate.

The indications for ACDF are broad because of the ability to address most anterior disorders. Indications include cervical stenosis, foraminal stenosis (unilateral or bilateral), disc herniation, soft disc herniation, instability, and cervical spondylosis.

The indications for posterior cervical foraminotomy are narrower. PCF is mostly reserved for 1-level or 2-level unilateral radiculopathy. In addition, this technique is best for bony foraminal stenosis or soft disc herniations that are foraminal or with paracentral disc herniations with the apex lateral to the lateral edge of the spinal cord.

The indications for cervical arthroplasty continue to evolve as further randomized investigational device exemption studies conclude. At present, the indication is for 1-level and some 2-level myelopathic or radiculopathy cervical disease.

APPROACH TO SURGICAL DECISION MAKING

In determining the surgical options, the contributing disorder must be understood. Degenerative cervical spine disorder is often a spectrum of disease that can ultimately manifest with HNP. Therefore, it is likely that even with a clear soft disc herniation there will be some degree of cervical spondylotic disease as well. It is important to evaluate how this may be contributing to symptoms when determining the appropriate management and intervention for these patients. One epidemiologic study found that only 21.9% of patients with cervical radiculopathy have isolated disc herniation, whereas 68.4% had foraminal spondylosis alone or in combination with disc hernaition.[11–14]

Classifying the disc herniation into the following categories helps with decision making about the surgical approach: central disc herniation, paracentral disc herniation, and foraminal disc herniation (**Fig. 1**).

In addition, it is important to establish the degree of contributing spondylotic disease. If there is significant foraminal or central osteophytic disease, this may limit the surgical options. If there is concern for instability, this should be evaluated with flexion-extension radiographs.

In addition, the patient's clinical presentation is of paramount importance. The clinician must determine whether the symptoms and physical examination are most consistent with myelopathy, radiculopathy, or myeloradiculopathy. It is also helpful to assess for the presence and degree of axial neck pain. With this information, a surgical approach can be planned.

Table 1 presents an aid for surgical decision making with soft disc herniation. As with any decision in spine surgery, it is important to consider all patient-related factors in determining the best surgical decision for the patient. **Table 1** does not include factors that may significantly alter surgical decision making, including patient age, instability, prior surgical interventions, alignment, adjacent-segment disease, and bone quality. In general, if patients can be effectively treated with motion-preserving techniques (CTDR, PCF) these options should be presented to the patient. ACDF remains the workhorse approach because of its ability to address numerous underlying disorders, such as advanced spondylosis and multiple levels, in addition to soft disc herniation. Therefore, ACDF can be used for disc herniation over multiple levels (>2 levels) with or without axial neck pain, despite underlying kyphosis or advanced facet disease. CTDR is ideally suited for central and paracentral soft disc herniation, with or without neck pain, over 1 or 2 levels without significant facet disease or sagittal imbalance. PCF is ideally indicated for unilateral radiculopathy caused by bony foraminal stenosis or foraminal disc herniation without significant central stenosis or prominent axial neck pain.

ADJACENT-SEGMENT DISEASE

Understanding adjacent-segment diseases is essential when discussing ACDF, PCF, and CTDR. Theoretically, motion-preserving procedures

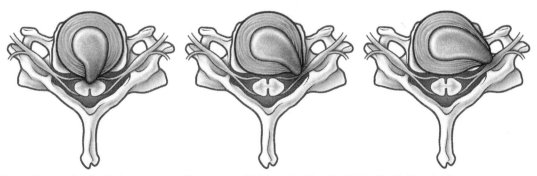

Fig. 1. Types of soft disc herniations. (Copyright of Atrium Health, Charlotte, North Carolina.)

Table 1
Surgical decision making for cervical soft disc herniation

| | | Soft Disc Herniation Location[a] | | |
		Foraminal	Central	Paracentral
Spondylosis Location	None	PCF[c]	CTDR[c]	CTDR[c]
		CTDR	ACDF	PCF[b]
		ACDF		ACDF
	Foraminal	PCF[c]	ACDF[c]	PCF
		ACDF	CTDR	ACDF[c]
		CTDR		CTDR
	Central	ACDF[c]	ACDF[c]	ACDF[c]
		CTDR	CTDR	CTDR

[a] PCF is contraindicated regardless of the location of the soft disc herniation in the setting of significant myelopathy or instability.
[b] If soft disc herniation apex is lateral to the thecal sac.
[c] Indicates an ideal indication.

reduce accelerated degeneration of adjacent segments that occur with fusion. Adjacent-segment degeneration is defined as new degenerative radiographic findings at an adjacent level. When these radiographic findings are associated with clinical symptoms, this is referred to as adjacent-segment disease. In addition, adjacent-segment reoperation refers to patients that require surgical intervention at the adjacent level.

It is important to understand that there is a natural history to the presence of adjacent-segment disease, even in the absence of surgical intervention. Several studies have described this phenomenon, which is an important concept when understanding rates of adjacent-segment disease. Matsumoto and colleagues[15] described a rate of adjacent segment in an asymptomatic population in their 20s and more than 60 years of age. They found that 17% of men and 13% of women in their 20s showed degenerative changes on MRI. This number increased to 86% and 89% of men and women respectively more than the age of 60 years. In addition, Gore[16] performed a 10-year observation of 159 asymptomatic patients with cervical radiographs. Seventy-two (45.2%) of the participants had degenerative findings on their initial radiographs. At 10-year follow-up, 70 (97.2%) of the 72 participants had progression of their degenerative findings. This study shows a clear natural history of the progression of adjacent-segment disease in the absence of surgical intervention. In addition, the degree of adjacent-segment disease may be affected by which levels undergo surgical intervention.

ACDF results in fusion across the disc space and loss of motion across the vertebral segment, which places increased stress on adjacent segments. It is theorized that there is a higher rate of adjacent-segment disease in ACDF because of this. Several biomechanical studies have shown that adjacent-level disc space and structures incur increased stress as a result of an adjacent fused segment.[21,22] There are several studies that have attempted to determine the long-term rates of Adjacent segment disease (ASD) in ACDF. This condition has been reported to occur at an annual rate of 1.3% to 4.5% in ACDF.[23–25]

The landmark study by Hilibrand and colleagues[26] is often cited when referencing adjacent-segment disease in ACDF. This study consisted of 374 patients followed for 10 years after ACDF. Adjacent-segment disease was defined as new radicular or myelopathy symptoms referable to an adjacent level on 2 consecutive office visits. This study reported an annual incidence of 2.9% per year over the 10-year period. However, only 27 patients had an adjacent-level surgery in the 10-year period for a total annual adjacent-level reoperation rate of 0.7% per year.

Motion-preserving techniques such as posterior cervical laminoforaminotomy and cervical arthroplasty are intended to preserve physiologic motion. This outcome theoretically reduces adjacent-level stresses and development of adjacent-segment disease. Wigfield and colleagues[27] showed reduced stress of the adjacent-level annulus in cadaveric specimens with artificial disc compared with ACDF.

When discussing adjacent-segment disease, the rate of adjacent-segment reoperation is the most objective and most clinically relevant outcome measure. The rate of adjacent-segment reoperation as described by Hilibrand and colleagues[26] may be as low as 0.7% per year in the ACDF population. As a result, the cervical arthroplasty trials will require long-term follow-up in order to show any significant effect in reducing reoperation rate. Many investigational device exemption studies are beginning to reach the 5-year and 10-year follow-up marks. Zigler and colleagues[28] reported 5-year follow-up results on ProDisc C, showing significantly lower rates of reoperation in the arthroplasty group than in the ACDF control group (2.9% vs 11.3%). Burkus and colleagues[29] presented 7-year follow-up on Prestige ST, showing a lower adjacent-segment reoperation rate in arthroplasty compared with ACDF (4.6% vs 11.9%). Lavelle and colleagues[30] reported on the 10-year outcome of the BRYAN artificial disc, showing reduced adjacent-segment reoperation rates compared with ACDF (9.7% vs 15.8%).

Similarly, cervical laminoforaminotomy results obtained over many years confirm much lower rates of adjacent-level disease and same-level disease. Henderson and colleagues[7] in 736 patients found an adjacent-level recurrence rate of 5.2% and same-level rate of 3.3%. More recently, Clarke and colleagues[31] reviewed 303 patients and found an adjacent-level rate of 6.7% (0.7% per year) and same-segment rate of 5% at 10 years.

The rates of same-segment and adjacent-segment disease for posterior cervical foraminotomy are more than half the rates for anterior decompression and fusion. Many spine surgeons are not trained to do posterior laminoforaminotomy in any form, open or minimally invasive. It should be the goal of all well-rounded spine surgeons to be skilled at both anterior and posterior approaches to treat radiculopathy, and then to select the most appropriate for the patient's individual disorder.

COMMON COMPLICATIONS AND AVOIDANCE

Anterior and posterior approaches to the treatment of degenerative cervical spine disorder generally have low complication rates. Despite this, the anterior approach has significant potential approach-related morbidities as a result of the number of adjacent neck structures in the operative corridor. These complications are shared by both ACDF and CTDR and can be minimized by proper blunt and sharp dissection technique in the correct anatomic planes. **Table 2** presents a summary of anterior cervical approach complication rates.

In addition to the anterior approach complications presented, there are additional complications unique to CTDR. These complications include device expulsion/dislocation/subsidence as well as focal kyphosis and heterotopic

Table 2
Summary of anterior cervical spine complication rates

Complication	Rate (%)
Airway compromise	0.6–1.6
Esophageal perforation	0–3.4
Dysphagia	47–50
Vascular injuries	0.7–1.4
Dural tears, cerebrospinal fluid leak	0–18
Infection	0.2–1.6
Implant malposition, pullout	0.085–7
Hypoglossal nerve injury	0.01
Superior laryngeal nerve injury	0–1.25

ossification (HO), which has questionable clinical significance. Attention to proper surgical technique can help minimize these complications, including use of intraoperative fluoroscopy for meticulous midline verification and proper device sizing. Symmetric posterior disc release should be obtained with resection of the posterior longitudinal ligament and proximal bilateral uncovertebral joints. Drilling should be avoided when possible, and the bony endplates should be respected, which limits HO and subsidence. Proper device sizing is important because an oversized implant limits motion and places

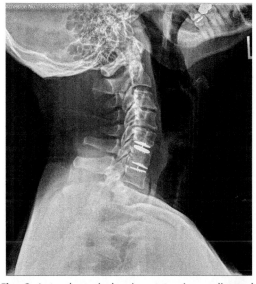

Fig. 2. Lateral cervical spine extension radiograph showing history of prior C5-C6, C6-C7 artificial disc replacement.

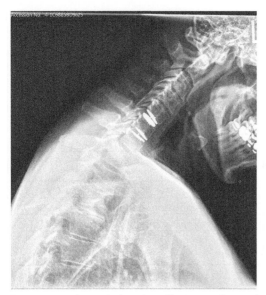

Fig. 3. Lateral cervical spine flexion radiograph showing history of prior C5-C6, C6-C7 artificial disc replacement.

increased stresses on the facet joints. Maximal endplate coverage with the device also limits HO and subsidence.

The MELF has additional complication risks unique to the posterior approach. There is typically increased muscle morbidity and bleeding compared with the anterior approach. These complications can be minimized by using a minimally invasive, sitting position, muscle-splitting approach. During positioning, avoid overflexion, which may make the neural elements vulnerable

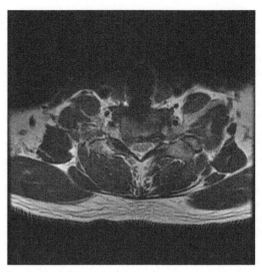

Fig. 5. Axial T2 cervical MRI showing a right C7-T1 foraminal disc herniation.

to damage from inadvertent advancement of the Kirschner wire (K-wire) or dilators between the lamina. Skin incision should be carried deep to the subcutaneous fascia, allowing placement of K-wire and dilators with minimal resistance, minimizing the risk of inadvertent advancement. Tubular retractor should be centered over the disc space in the cephalad-caudal direction (as seen on lateral fluoroscopy). Lamina-facet junction should be positioned one-third of the way from the medial border of the tubular retractor (as seen by direct visualization). The pedicle is the critical anatomic landmark, and its medial border should be drilled flush with the vertebral body to minimize

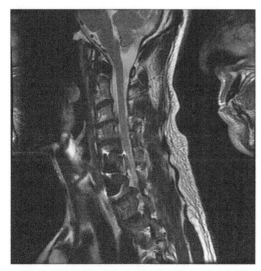

Fig. 4. Sagittal T2 cervical MRI showing a right C7-T1 foraminal disc herniation.

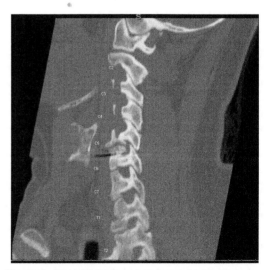

Fig. 6. Sagittal CT C spine showing right C5-C6 neuroforaminal stenosis.

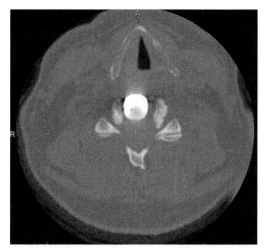

Fig. 7. Axial CT C spine showing right C5-C6 neuroforaminal stenosis.

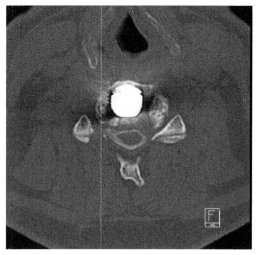

Fig. 9. Axial CT C spine myelogram showing postoperative decompression of right C5-C6 foramen.

neural retraction and postoperative radicular pain or neurologic deficit.

CASE STUDY A

A 53-year-old man with a prior history of C5-C6, C6-C7 CTDR 4 years earlier now presents with new symptoms of neck and right arm pain that radiates to his elbow and fourth and fifth digits of his hand. Physical examination findings included 4+/5 grip strength on the right and positive Spurling test. He underwent updated cervical spine radiographs, which reveal prior C5-C6, C6-C7 artificial disc in good position with preserved motion (**Figs. 2** and **3**). MRI of cervical spine revealed a right C7-T1 foraminal disc herniation with severe

foraminal stenosis (**Figs. 4** and **5**). He failed conservative therapy, including physical therapy, nonsteroidal antiinflammatory drugs, and epidural steroid injection. He ultimately was offered a right C7-T1 minimally invasive endoscopic laminoforaminotomy. This procedure was performed in an ambulatory surgery center with an operative time of 28 minutes, and the patient was discharged home 2 hours postoperatively with complete resolution of his symptoms.

CASE STUDY B

A 59-year-old man with a prior history of C5-C6 CTDR 2 years earlier. He now presents with right

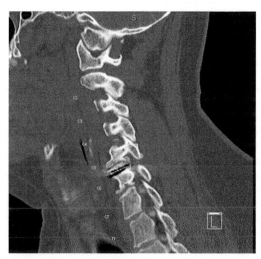

Fig. 8. Sagittal CT C spine myelogram showing postoperative decompression of Right C5-C6 foramen.

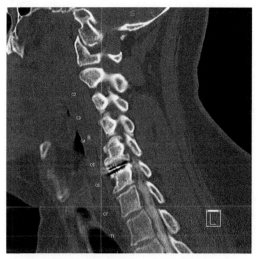

Fig. 10. Sagittal CT C spine myelogram showing severe right C4-C5 foraminal stenosis.

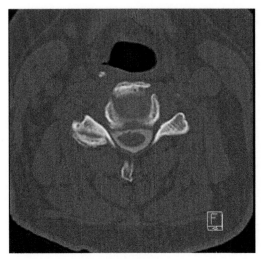

Fig. 11. Axial CT C spine myelogram showing severe right C4-C5 foraminal stenosis.

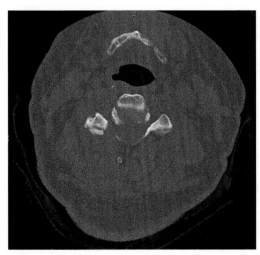

Fig. 13. Axial CT C spine showing decompressed right C4-C5 foramen postoperatively.

neck and arm pain in his right thumb and first finger. Computed tomography (CT) cervical spine (C spine) revealed severe bony foraminal stenosis on the right at C5 to C6 at the index level (**Figs. 6** and **7**). He received a right-sided C5-C6 nerve root block, which provided good improvement of his symptoms temporarily before returning. He then underwent a right C5-C6 minimally invasive endoscopic laminoforaminotomy. This procedure was performed in an ambulatory surgery center with a 21-minute operative time. The patient was discharged home 2 hours postoperatively. He had resolution

of his radicular symptoms. He subsequently returned after his 1-year follow-up with new right arm symptoms, now radiating into his right shoulder and forearm. He underwent CT myelogram of his cervical spine, which revealed severe right C4-C5 foraminal stenosis, and adequate decompression of his prior right-sided C5-C6 foraminotomy site (**Figs. 8–11**). He received 2 separate right C4-C5 nerve root blocks, which provided him with 80% relief with eventual return of his symptoms. He then underwent a right C4-C5 minimally invasive endoscopic laminoforaminotomy. This procedure was performed in an ambulatory surgery center with a 31-minute operative time. The patient was discharge home 2 hours after surgery. This procedure resulted in resolution of his symptoms. Postoperative CT C spine reveals decompression of the R C4-C5 foramen (**Figs. 12** and **13**).

SUMMARY

ACDF, CTDR, and PCF are effective procedures for the treatment of a broad range of degenerative cervical disorders. In particular, these procedures are extremely effective in the treatment of cervical radiculopathy. Additional considerations of minimally invasive technique, outpatient setting, motion preservation, and adjacent-segment disease should be taken into consideration when formulating a surgical plan. It should be the goal of all well-rounded spine surgeons to be skilled at both anterior and posterior approaches to treat radiculopathy, and then to select the most appropriate for the patient's individual disorder.

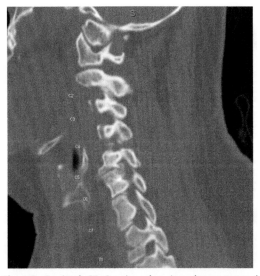

Fig. 12. Sagittal CT C spine showing decompressed right C4-C5 foramen postoperatively.

CLINICS CARE POINTS

- ACDF has satisfactory results in 90% to 95% of patients.

- The indications for CTDR are radiculopathy with 1-level or 2-level cervical soft disc herniation caused by central or paracentral disc herniation.

- PCF was first popularized by Spurling, Scoville, and Frykholm in the 1950s. The minimally invasive cervical microendoscopic laminoforaminotomy technique was described by Adamson[29] in 2001.

- The landmark study by Hilibrand and colleagues[22] is often cited when referencing adjacent-segment disease in ACDF. This study consisted of 374 patients followed for 10 years after ACDF. Adjacent-segment disease was defined as new radicular or myelopathy symptoms referable to an adjacent level on 2 consecutive office visits. This study reported an annual incidence of 2.9% per year over the 10-year period.

- Many CTDR investigational device exemption studies are beginning to reach the 5-year and 10-year follow-up marks. Zigler and colleagues[24] reported 5-year follow-up results on ProDisc C, showing significantly lower rates of reoperation in the arthroplasty group than in the ACDF control group (2.9% vs 11.3%). Burkus and colleagues[25] presented 7-year follow-up on Prestige ST, showing a lower adjacent-segment reoperation rate in arthroplasty compared with ACDF (4.6% vs 11.9%). Lavelle and colleagues[26] reported on the 10-year outcome of BRYAN artificial disc, showing reduced adjacent-segment reoperation rates compared with ACDF (9.7% vs 15.8%).

DISCLOSURES

The authors have nothing to disclose.

REFERENCES

1. Stookey B. Compression of the spinal cord due to ventral extradural cervical chondromas: diagnosis and surgical treatment. J Nerv Ment Dis. 1928;20:275-291.
2. Frykholm R. Deformities of dural pouches and strictures of dural sheaths in the cervical region producing nerve-root compression; a contribution to the etiology and operative treatment of brachial neuralgia. J Neurosurg 1947;4(5):403–13.
3. Murphey F, Simmons JC. Ruptured cervical disc. Experience with 250 cases. Am Surg 1966;32(2):83–8.
4. Cloward RB. The anterior approach for removal of ruptured cervical disks. J Neurosurg 1958;15(6):602–17.
5. Robinson RA, Smith GW. Anterolateral disc removal and interbody fusion for cervical disc syndrome. Bull Johns Hopkins Hosp 1955;96:223–4.
6. Zeidman SM, Ducker TB. Posterior cervical laminoforaminotomy for radiculopathy: review of 172 cases. Neurosurgery 1993;33(3):356–62.
7. Henderson CM, Hennessy RG, Shuey HM, et al. Posterior-lateral foraminotomy as an exclusive operative technique for cervical radiculopathy: a review of 846 consecutively operated cases. Neurosurgery 1983;13(5):504–12.
8. Frykholm, R. (1951). Cervical root compression resulting from disc degeneration and root sleeve fibrosis. Acta Chir Scand, 160, 1-149.
9. Cummins BH, Robertson JT, Gill SS. Surgical experience with an implanted artificial cervical joint. J Neurosurg 1998 Jun;88(6):943–8.
10. Spurling RG, Scoville WB. Lateral rupture of the cervical intervertebral discs: a common cause of shoulder and arm pain. Gynecology and Obstetrics 1944;78:350–8.
11. Coric D, Cassis J, Carew JD, et al. Prospective study of cervical arthroplasty in 98 patients involved in 1 of 3 separate investigational device exemption studies from a single investigational site with a minimum 2-year follow-up. Clinical article. J Neurosurg Spine 2010;13(6):715–21.
12. Coric D, Nunley PD, Guyer RD, et al. Prospective, randomized, multicenter study of cervical arthroplasty: 269 patients from the Kineflex|C artificial disc investigational device exemption study with a minimum 2-year follow-up: clinical article. J Neurosurg Spine 2011;15(4):348–58.
13. Radcliff K, Coric D, Albert T. Five-year clinical results of cervical total disc replacement compared with anterior discectomy and fusion for treatment of 2-level symptomatic degenerative disc disease: a prospective, randomized, controlled, multicenter investigational device exemption clinical trial. J Neurosurg Spine 2016;25(2):213–24.
14. Zhang Y, Liang C, Tao Y, et al. Cervical total disc replacement is superior to anterior cervical decompression and fusion: a meta-analysis of prospective randomized controlled trials. PLoS One 2015;10(3):e0117826.
15. Matsumoto M, Fujimura Y, Suzuki N, et al. MRI of cervical intervertebral discs in asymptomatic subjects. J Bone Joint Surg Br 1998;80(1):19–24.

16. Gore DR. Roentgenographic findings in the cervical spine in asymptomatic persons: a ten-year follow-up. Spine 2001;26(22):2463–6.

17. Foley KT. Microendoscopic discectomy. Tech Neurosurg 1997;3:301–7.

18. Adamson TE. Microendoscopic posterior cervical laminoforaminotomy for unilateral radiculopathy: results of a new technique in 100 cases. J Neurosurg 2001;95(1 Suppl):51–7.

19. Coric D, Adamson T. Minimally invasive cervical microendoscopic laminoforaminotomy. Neurosurg Focus 2008;25(2):E2.

20. Hilton DL. Minimally invasive tubular access for posterior cervical foraminotomy with three-dimensional microscopic visualization and localization with anterior/posterior imaging. Spine J 2007; 7(2):154–8.

21. Eck JC, Humphreys SC, Lim T-H, et al. Biomechanical study on the effect of cervical spine fusion on adjacent-level intradiscal pressure and segmental motion. Spine 2002;27(22):2431–4.

22. Lopez-Espina CG, Amirouche F, Havalad V. Multilevel cervical fusion and its effect on disc degeneration and osteophyte formation. Spine 2006;31(9): 972–8.

23. Bohlman HH, Emery SE, Goodfellow DB, et al. Robinson anterior cervical discectomy and arthrodesis for cervical radiculopathy. Long-term follow-up of one hundred and twenty-two patients. J Bone Joint Surg Am 1993;75(9):1298–307.

24. Gore DR, Sepic SB. Anterior discectomy and fusion for painful cervical disc disease. A report of 50 patients with an average follow-up of 21 years. Spine 1998;23(19):2047–51.

25. Cauthen JC, Kinard RE, Vogler JB, et al. Outcome analysis of noninstrumented anterior cervical discectomy and interbody fusion in 348 patients. Spine 1998;23(2):188–92.

26. Hilibrand AS, Carlson GD, Palumbo MA, et al. Radiculopathy and myelopathy at segments adjacent to the site of a previous anterior cervical arthrodesis. J Bone Joint Surg Am 1999;81(4):519–28.

27. Wigfield CC, Skrzypiec D, Jackowski A, et al. Internal stress distribution in cervical intervertebral discs: the influence of an artificial cervical joint and simulated anterior interbody fusion. J Spinal Disord Tech 2003;16(5):441–9.

28. Zigler JE, Delamarter R, Murrey D, et al. ProDisc-C and anterior cervical discectomy and fusion as surgical treatment for single-level cervical symptomatic degenerative disc disease: five-year results of a Food and Drug Administration study. Spine 2013; 38(3):203–9.

29. Burkus JK, Traynelis VC, Haid RW, et al. Clinical and radiographic analysis of an artificial cervical disc: 7-year follow-up from the Prestige prospective randomized controlled clinical trial: Clinical article. J Neurosurg Spine 2014;21(4):516–28.

30. Lavelle WF, Riew KD, Levi AD, et al. Ten-year outcomes of cervical disc replacement with the BRYAN cervical disc: results from a prospective, randomized, controlled clinical trial. Spine 2019;44(9): 601–8.

31. Clarke MJ, Ecker RD, Krauss WE, et al. Same-segment and adjacent-segment disease following posterior cervical foraminotomy. J Neurosurg Spine 2007;6(1):5–9.

Biomechanics of Cervical Disc Arthroplasty Devices

Avinash G. Patwardhan, PhD[a,b,*], Robert M. Havey, MS[a]

KEYWORDS

• Cervical spine • Cervical disc arthroplasty • Total disc replacement • Biomechanics

KEY POINTS

- Prosthesis design has an influence on the quantity and quality of postoperative motion after cervical disc arthroplasty (CDA).
- Prostheses that allow translation independent of rotation allow the spinal anatomy to dictate the segmental motion.
- A 6-degrees-of-freedom disc prosthesis may be best equipped to achieve the intended function of CDA.
- A disc prosthesis with built-in resistance to angular and translational motion may have an advantage in restoring stability to a hypermobile segment without eliminating motion.
- The location and orientation of axes of rotation in flexion-extension, lateral bending and axial rotation influence the loading of facet and uncovertebral joints and soft-tissues.

INTRODUCTION

Historically, anterior cervical discectomy and fusion (ACDF) has been used widely to treat symptomatic cervical spondylosis.[1–4] Several clinical studies have shown cervical disc arthroplasty (CDA) to be a viable alternative to ACDF for the treatment of radiculopathy and myelopathy.[5–19] The proposed advantages of disc arthroplasty are based on the premise that preservation of physiologic motions and load sharing at the treated level leads to longevity of the facet joints at the index level and mitigates the risk of adjacent segment degeneration.

The goal of CDA is to restore normal biomechanical function to the diseased cervical spine segment, thereby allowing it to support the physiologic loads and motions of daily activities without pain. The design features of cervical disc prostheses influence their ability to restore physiologic range of motion (ROM) and load sharing between the facets and anterior column. This article expands on these concepts using data from the literature and on the basis of the authors' experience in assessing the biomechanical function of different artificial disc prostheses.

CERVICAL DISC PROSTHESES DESIGNS
Constrained, Unconstrained, and Semiconstrained—What Do These Terms Mean?

The discussion in the literature regarding the design of artificial disc prostheses is complicated by the ambiguity surrounding the use of terms, such as *constrained, unconstrained,* and *semiconstrained*. In biomechanics (and kinematics in particular), the term, *constraint*, refers to a limit on the number of kinematic degrees of freedom (DOFs) (ie, the number of independent motion components) an object has during its motion in 3-dimensional (3-D) space. An object with 0 constraints on its movement is said to have unconstrained motion having 6 DOFs in 3-D space, which is to say it can rotate independently about 3 orthogonal axes and translate independently

[a] Musculoskeletal Biomechanics Laboratory, Edward Hines, Jr. VA Hospital, PO Box 5000, Hines, IL, 60141 USA;
[b] Department of Orthopedic Surgery and Rehabilitation, Loyola University Medical Center, 2160 South First Avenue, Maywood, IL 60153, USA
* Corresponding author.
E-mail address: apatwar@lumc.edu

Neurosurg Clin N Am 32 (2021) 493–504
https://doi.org/10.1016/j.nec.2021.05.008
1042-3680/21/Published by Elsevier Inc.

along these 3 axes. All 6 components of motion are independently possible; for example, translational motion of the object can occur without the need for rotation. The discussion of DOFs of a prosthesis is relevant because it has a bearing on the ability of the prosthesis to work in concert with the remaining soft issue structures, facet joints, and uncovertebral joints after CDA.

Sears and colleagues[20] suggested that when prostheses offer intrinsic resistance (stiffness) against bending or translational motions, they should be regarded as restrained, not constrained. A restrained prosthesis should not be confused with one that has built-in physical stops for limiting translational or angular motions allowed by the prosthesis.

Classification of Cervical Disc Prosthesis Designs

Artificial cervical disc prostheses have been classified over the years using different criteria. Sears and colleagues[20] used kinematic DOFs and constraints to classify various cervical and lumbar disc prostheses. Büttner-Janz[21] classified various prostheses based on the number of articulating components that form joints (bearings) to produce motion within the prosthesis. This article provides a discussion of the DOFs afforded by various disc prosthesis designs within the different categories that are based on the number of articulating components.

Three-component cervical disc prostheses

The kinematic DOFs of a disc prosthesis are determined by the nature of articulation of the bearing surfaces of the prosthesis. A disc prosthesis with 3 components can have 2 articulating bearings (joints) (**Fig. 1**). For example, a prosthesis with an incompressible, biconvex core has 2 DOFs in both the sagittal and coronal planes. The mobile core allows independent rotation in each plane without the need for translation and a limited amount of translation between the vertebrae in each plane independent of the rotation. In the axial plane, the prosthesis has 1 additional DOF that is unaccounted for in the sagittal plane or coronal plane motions, namely, axial rotation. Thus, a 3-component prosthesis with a biconvex mobile core allows 3 independent angular motions (flexion-extension [FE], lateral bending, and axial rotation), along with 2 independent translations (along anterior-posterior and lateral directions), for a total of 5 DOFs. The only missing DOF is the ability to compress along the superior-inferior axis of the disc. Some examples of this prosthesis design include the Charité lumbar disc (see **Fig. 1**A),[22] the Kineflex|C (Spinal Motion, Mountain View, CA, USA),[15] and

the recently approved Simplify cervical disc (see **Fig. 1**B).[23]

Another example of a prosthesis with 3 articulating components with 2 bearings is the Mobi-C cervical artificial disc (see **Fig. 1**C). The bearing (joint) formed by the mobile core with the superior prosthetic end plate is spherical, which allows 3 independent angular motions. The core forms a planar bearing with the inferior prosthetic end plate, which allows translational motions (up to 1.25 mm) in the sagittal and coronal planes. The Mobi-C prosthesis has a total of 5 DOFs in 3-D space. The only missing DOF is the ability to compress along the superior-inferior axis of the disc.

The Secure-C disc prosthesis has a mobile core that forms a spherical (ball-and-socket) bearing with the superior prosthetic end plate and a cylindrical bearing with the inferior prosthetic end plate with the long axis of the cylinder aligned in the coronal plane (see **Fig. 1**D). The cylindrical and spherical joints both allow FE motions and, therefore, the upper vertebra can translate a small amount in the anterior-posterior direction without the need to undergo FE angular motion. As a result, in the sagittal plane, the prosthesis allows motion with 2 kinematic DOFs. In the coronal plane, the angular motion in lateral bending is allowed only at the superior spherical joint. Thus, the prosthesis functions as a 2-component prosthesis in this plane. The Secure-C prosthesis allows 3 independent angular motions (FE, lateral bending, and axial rotation) and 1 independent translation along the anterior-posterior direction, yielding a total of 4 DOFs. No translation motion is allowed along the superior-inferior direction or in the lateral direction in the coronal plane.

Two-component cervical disc prostheses

Artificial cervical disc prostheses with 2 functional components that articulate to produce motion in the prosthesis can have different kinematic DOFs depending on the type of bearing (joint). A prosthesis with 2 articulating components with 1 spherical bearing (ball-and-socket joint) has 3 DOFs because it can allow only 3 independent angular motions; namely, FE, lateral bending, and axial rotation. No translational motion between the 2 components is possible if the conformal bearing surfaces remain fully in contact during the arc of motion. Some examples of this class of cervical disc prostheses include the Pro-Disc-C,[16] DePuy Discover,[24] and porous coated motion (PCM) discs[10] (**Fig. 2**A–C).

Other examples of joints that prostheses with 2 articulating components form include a saddle joint, a ball-and-trough joint, and noncongruent ball-and-socket joints. A saddle joint allows independent angular motions in 2 orthogonal planes; for example,

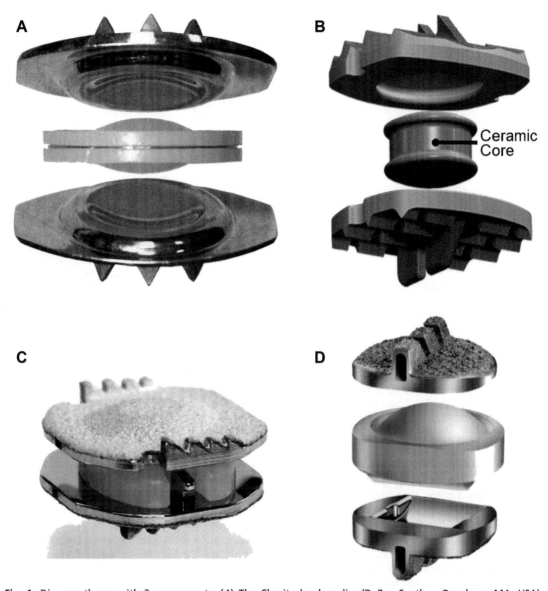

Fig. 1. Disc prostheses with 3 components. (*A*) The Charite lumbar disc (DePuy Synthes, Raynham, MA, USA), which includes 2 metal end plates and a biconvex mobile core that articulate in 2 spherical bearings (ball-and-socket joints). (*B*) The Simplify cervical disc prosthesis, also with a biconvex mobile core (Nuvasive, San Diego, CA, USA). (*C*) Mobi-C cervical artificial disc (Zimmer Biomet, Warsaw, IN, USA). The bearing formed by the mobile core with the superior prosthetic end plate is spherical. The core forms a planar bearing with the inferior prosthetic end plate. (*D*) The Secure-C (Globus Medical, Audubon, PA, USA) disc prosthesis, which has a mobile core that forms a spherical (ball-and-socket) bearing with the superior prosthetic end plate and a cylindrical bearing with the inferior prosthetic end plate with the long axis of the cylinder aligned in the coronal plane. (Images reprinted from Patwardhan AG, Havey RM. Biomechanics of Cervical Disc Arthroplasty–A Review of Concepts and Current Technology. *Int J Spine Surg*. 2020;14(s2):S14-S28. https://doi.org/10.14444/7087. Copyright (c) 2020 International Society for the Advancement of Spine Surgery.[42])

FE and lateral bending. Therefore, a prosthesis with an articulating saddle joint (for example, the Cervi-Core disc [**Fig. 2**D]) has 2 DOFs.[25]

A ball-and-trough articulation, such as in the Prestige disc (**Fig. 2**E), allows 3 independent angular motions (FE, lateral bending, and axial rotation) and translation independent of FE motion in the sagittal plane.[18] Therefore, a prosthesis with a ball-and-trough articulation, such as the Prestige LP or Prestige ST, has 4 DOFs.

A recent addition to the category of 2-component prostheses is a design with a 3-lobe

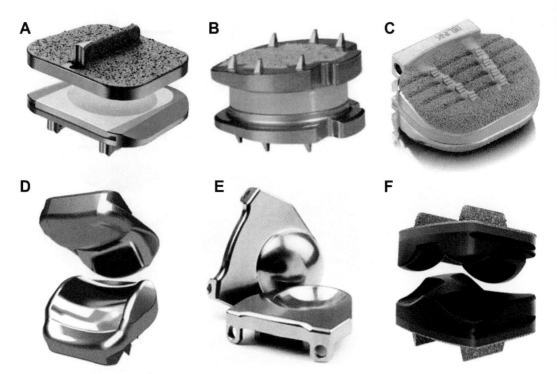

Fig. 2. Prostheses with 2 articulating components. (*A*) ProDisc-C (Centinel Spine, West Chester, PA, USA), (*B*) Discover (DePuy Synthes, Raynham, MA, USA), (*C*) PCM (Nuvasive, San Diego, CA, USA), (*D*) Cervicore (Stryker, Kalamazoo, MI, USA), (*E*) Prestige LP (Medtronic, Memphis TN, USA), and (*F*) Triadyme-C (Dymicron, Orem, UT, USA). (Images reprinted from Patwardhan AG, Havey RM. Biomechanics of Cervical Disc Arthroplasty–A Review of Concepts and Current Technology. *Int J Spine Surg*. 2020;14(s2):S14-S28. https://doi.org/10.14444/7087. Copyright (c) 2020 International Society for the Advancement of Spine Surgery.[42])

articulation in which the mating surfaces are noncongruent (Triadyme-C [**Fig. 2**F]). The radii of the lobes are smaller than the corresponding pockets. Because of this design, load transfer from the superior lobes to the inferior pockets occurs over a small surface area, resulting in very-high-contact stresses. Industrial polycrystalline diamond, specially formulated and processed for biocompatibility, is used to resist the high-contact stresses. This prosthesis allows 3 primary rotations, coupled with anterior-posterior and medial-lateral translations.[26] The device is noncompressible with 3 independent DOFs.

Nonarticulating cervical disc prostheses

Nonarticulating cervical disc prosthesis designs include viscoelastic compressible cores; for example, a polycarbonate polyurethane core that allows compression or shortening of the disc prosthesis height. This component of motion, which was missing in the incompressible designs, allows the disc to have all 6 kinematic DOFs. Some examples of this design include the Bryan,[14] the M6-C disc,[27] the Rhine disc,[28] and the CP-ESP disc[29] (**Fig. 3**).

In addition to the kinematic DOFs, the ability of the prosthesis to offer a built-in or inherent resistance to angular and translational motions is an important design feature that affects its ability to restore physiologic motion as well as stability, both of which are the functional goals of a cervical disc prosthesis. Prostheses with viscoelastic compressible cores offer some amount of inherent resistance (stiffness) to angular and translational motions, depending on the dimensions of the core, stiffness of the polymer material, and its fixation to the prosthetic end plates. Of the discs with a viscoelastic compressible core, the M6-C disc incorporates additional feature; namely, an artificial annulus made of polyethylene fibers woven through holes in the 2 inner metal end plates of the disc. The fiber annulus provides added bending stiffness to the disc, a feature that can be important for restoring bending stiffness to a hypermobile segment.

INFLUENCE OF PROSTHESIS DESIGN ON MOTION AFTER DISC REPLACEMENT
Effect of Prosthesis Design on Range of Motion

The authors compared the ROM of cervical segments implanted with different designs of disc

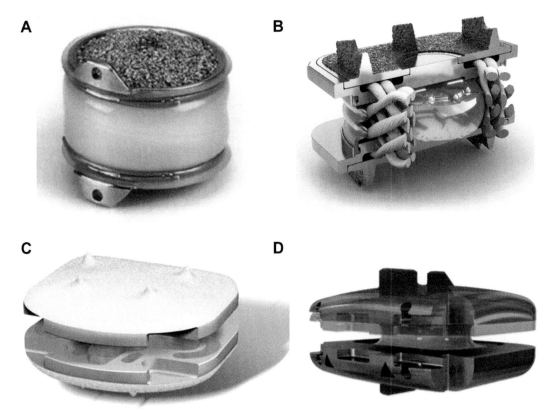

Fig. 3. A class of nonarticulating discs with compressible cores. (*A*) Bryan disc (Medtronic, Memphis TN, USA), (*B*) M6-C disc (Orthofix Medical Inc, Lewisville, TX, USA), (*C*) CP-ESP disc (Spine Innovations, Heimsbrunn, France), and (*D*) Rhine disc (Stryker, Kalamazoo, MI, USA). (Images reprinted from Patwardhan AG, Havey RM. Biomechanics of Cervical Disc Arthroplasty–A Review of Concepts and Current Technology. *Int J Spine Surg*. 2020;14(s2):S14-S28. https://doi.org/10.14444/7087. Copyright (c) 2020 International Society for the Advancement of Spine Surgery.[42])

prostheses.[30] Disc prostheses of 3 design types were implanted: 2-component discs with a single spherical bearing, mobile core discs, and nonarticulating compressible core discs. All disc prostheses were implanted at either C5-6 or C6-7 with each prosthesis centered in the frontal plane and slightly posterior to the midline of the disc space in the sagittal plane.

All disc prostheses restored the ROM in FE to within the physiologic range reported in the literature (**Fig. 4**). The axial rotation and lateral bending ROMs were reduced after disc arthroplasty; this was true for fixed core discs, mobile core discs, and compressible core discs. The decrease in axial rotation and lateral bending motions after total disc replacement has been reported in previous biomechanical studies.[25,31–34] Guyer and colleagues[28] reported similar ROM results for the Rhine disc (6 DOFs elastic core design): in FE, ROM was restored to physiologic values; whereas, in lateral bending and axial rotation the ROM was reduced post-arthroplasty by 40% to 60%.

Clinical studies of ROM in lateral bending and axial rotation after cervical arthroplasty are not yet available.

Effect of Prosthesis Design on the Relationship Between Preoperative and Postoperative Motion

A CDA should restore physiologic motion while maintaining stability at the index segment. In a patient with limited mobility at the index segment, disc arthroplasty should restore normal physiologic motion. Conversely, if a motion segment is hypermobile, the prosthesis should restore stability by eliminating hypermobility. A study was performed to investigate the influence of prosthesis design on the relationship between preoperative and postoperative ROM after CDA. The relationships between FE motions of cervical segments before and after disc replacement were investigated using 7 different cervical disc prostheses classified into 3 design groups: (1) discs with a single spherical bearing Advent (Blackstone Medical,

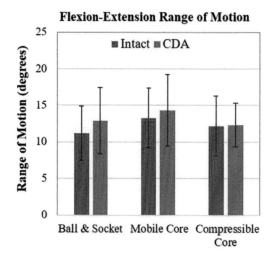

Fig. 4. FE-ROM intact and after CDA using 3 different CDA designs: single spherical bearing (ball-and-socket), mobile core, and compressible core. ROM is from C5-6 and C6-7 segments under 150 N of compressive preload.

Prodisc-C, Discover, and PCM); (2) mobile core discs (Mobi-C, Kineflex|C); and (3) restrained compressible core disc (M6-C).[35,36]

In segments reconstructed using single spherical bearing disc prostheses, the FE-ROM after disc arthroplasty was positively correlated with preoperative FE-ROM (R^2 = 0.66; P<.001) (**Fig. 5**A). Preoperative FE-ROM ranged from 5° to 22°, whereas motion after disc arthroplasty ranged from 2° to 23°.

In segments reconstructed using mobile core disc prostheses, the FE-ROM after disc arthroplasty was correlated positively with preoperative FE-ROM (R^2 = 0.20; P = .025) (**Fig. 5**B). Preoperative FE-ROM ranged from 6° to 21°, whereas, motion after disc arthroplasty ranged from 7° to 24°.

These results suggest that with both single spherical bearing discs and mobile core discs, segments with large preoperative mobility are expected to have large postoperative mobility. In contrast, in segments reconstructed using a restrained compressible core disc prosthesis, the postoperative FE-ROM was not correlated with preoperative FE-ROM (R^2 = 0.17; P = .12) (**Fig. 5**C). The lack of correlation means the preoperative ROM did not define the postoperative ROM. Preoperative FE-ROM ranged from 5° to 21°; whereas, motion after disc arthroplasty ranged 8° to 17°. This is beneficial when the goal is to reduce ROM of a hypermobile disc or increase ROM of a disc with low mobility.

These results suggest that the design features of cervical disc prostheses maybe matched to a patient's preoperative mobility to achieve the best postoperative outcomes of restoring physiologic motion while maintaining stability at the index segment.

Effect of Prosthesis Design on the Axes of Rotation of a Motion Segment

The axis of rotation in FE of the single spherical bearing (ball-and-socket joint) prosthesis passes through the center of curvature of the spherical bearing, which is located caudally in relation to the disc space (**Fig. 6**). Typically, the socket is implanted in the superior vertebra and the ball in the inferior vertebra of the segment. The center of the sphere would be the center of rotation (COR) for an arc of motion during which the bearing surfaces of the ball and socket remain fully in contact. The radius of the ball dictates the ratio of apparent translation experienced by the superior vertebra for every degree of angular motion. The larger the radius of the ball, the greater the apparent translation of the superior vertebra over

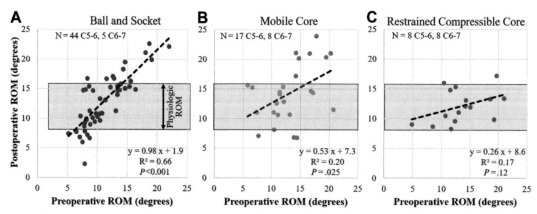

Fig. 5. Effect of preoperative ROM on postoperative ROM after CDA reconstruction (at C5-6 or C6-7) using 3 different CDA designs: (A) single spherical bearing (ball-and-socket), (B) mobile core, and (C) compressible core.

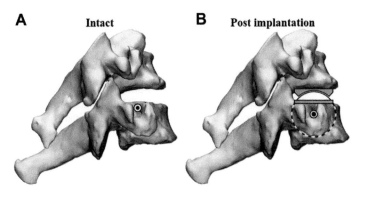

Fig. 6. FE axes of rotation in a C5-6 motion segment: (*A*) intact COR and (*B*) COR after CDA with a single spherical bearing prosthesis.

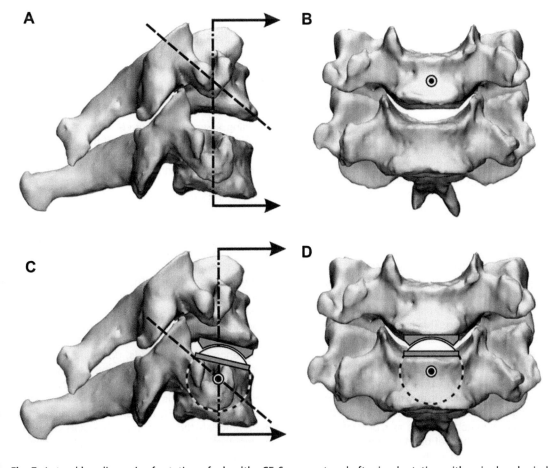

Fig. 7. Lateral bending axis of rotation of a healthy C5-6 segment and after implantation with a single spherical bearing prosthesis. (A) sagittal projection in a healthy segment (B) intersection of the lateral bending axis in the mid-coronal plane in a healthy segment (C) sagittal projection of the axis in a segment implanted with a single spherical bearing prosthesis and (D) intersection of the lateral bending axis in the mid-coronal plane after implantation with a single spherical bearing prosthesis.

the inferior.[20] The location of the ball relative to the disc space will influence the COR of the implanted segment, which will have an influence on the segmental motion, the amount of apparent translation of superior vertebra and stresses experienced by the soft tissues and facet joints.

A ball-and-trough articulation, such as in the Prestige prosthesis, uses a spherical dome implanted in the superior vertebra and the trough or elongated socket in the inferior vertebra. In this design, the ball can translate and rotate within the trough so the COR in FE is located distal to the inferior end plate of the intervertebral disc. Because of its ability to translate, the axis of rotation of the Prestige disc prosthesis is not fixed as in ball-and-socket designs. The location of the ball (or dome) in the superior vertebra as in the Prestige or Triadyme-C prostheses, instead of in the inferior vertebra as in a ball-and-socket designs, does not negatively affect the kinematics of segmental motion after disc arthroplasty.

In lateral bending, the axis of rotation of the native segment is in the cranial vertebra (**Fig. 7**A, B), whereas, the axis of rotation of a ball-and-socket single spherical bearing prosthesis, inherent to its design, is located well caudal to the location of the native axis (**Fig. 7**C, D). Therefore, this mismatch of lateral bending axes of rotation may contribute to limiting post-arthroplasty motion in lateral bending. Whereas a 6-DOFs compressible core disc, in theory, has the potential to adapt to the lateral bending axis of rotation of the native segment, the observed decrease in lateral bending motion of the implanted segment may be secondary to the inability to rotate about a more cranial axis of rotation for all prostheses designs.

In axial rotation, the native axis of rotation is inclined in the superior-posterior to inferior-anterior direction perpendicular to the facet surfaces and passing through the disc space. Thus, the mismatches between the axial rotation axes of the native disc and the prostheses are not as great as in lateral bending. This is reflected in a smaller decrease in overall axial rotation motion than in lateral bending motion after disc arthroplasty.

The mobile core design with 2 spherical bearings has the potential, in theory, to match the native axes of rotation in all 3 modes. The spherical bearing between the core and the upper end plate would allow matching of the axis of rotation in FE, whereas the spherical bearing between the core and the lower end plate would give an axis in lateral bending that is in the cranial vertebra, similar to the location of the lateral bending axis in the native segment. Yet, results of in vitro experiments showed the mobile core disc (Kineflex|C)

also decreased the lateral bending ROM at the implanted segment. Similar findings were seen in recent in vitro experiments with the Mobi-C mobile core prosthesis. This suggests the mobile core cannot fully reproduce the native axes of rotation or does not have the capacity to mimic the combined rotations and translations necessary to reproduce the motions of a native disc. Further experimental and clinical verification of this postulation is needed.

Effect of Prosthesis Design on Kinematic Signature

The applied moment versus segmental angular motion curve (kinematic signature) of a segment after CDA is a combined result of the bending stiffness of the disc prosthesis and the tensioning of the soft tissues, such as the remaining disc annulus, posterior ligaments, and facet capsules. A few studies[26,34,37–39] have reported the kinematic signature of cervical spine segments after CDA with prostheses of various designs and compared the signatures with those of healthy cervical spine segments (**Fig. 8**). Even though a disc prosthesis may lack built-in bending stiffness, the height of the prosthesis in relation to the native disc height and the location of the prosthesis COR can have the effect of recruiting the soft tissues to contribute enough stiffness to make the resulting kinematic signature resemble a healthy motion segment. This may be at the cost, however, of nonphysiologic strains induced in the ligaments, remaining annulus, and facet capsules.[20]

INFLUENCE OF PROSTHESIS DESIGN ON LOAD SHARING IN THE 3-JOINT COMPLEX

The location of the natural COR of a cervical segment in FE motion is correlated with the location and orientation of the facet surfaces relative to the mid-disc plane.[40] Therefore, in the presence of a mismatch between the locations of the prosthesis COR and the natural COR of a cervical segment, the ligaments and facet capsules could experience abnormal strains, and the facets may experience abnormal loads, upsetting the normal load-sharing characteristic of the cervical 3-joint complex. Another possible complication is that the bone-prosthesis interface may experience movement during FE motions of the segment to accommodate the mismatch in the COR locations.

Hypothetically, a disc prosthesis with a translational DOF, such as one provided by a 3-component disc prosthesis with a mobile core or the 2-component prosthesis with a ball moving in a trough, has the potential to allow the prosthesis motion to be guided by the facet joints in response to the external

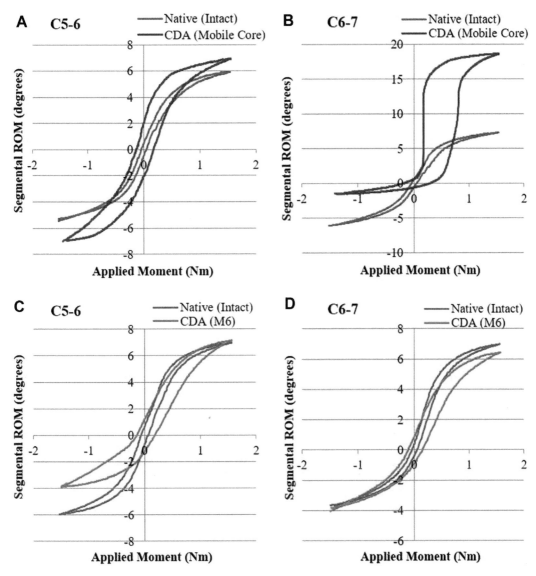

Fig. 8. Examples of kinematic signatures of cervical spine segments in FE: intact (native) and after CDA. (*A*) Good quality of motion after reconstruction using a mobile core disc prosthesis. (*B*) Sub-optimal motion showing excessive ROM of motion and low segment stiffness after mobile core prosthesis reconstruction, which may recruit increased muscle forces to stabilize the reconstructed segment.[41] (*C*) and (*D*) Motion after reconstruction using an M6-C disc prosthesis showing good range and quality of motion.

loads acting on the spine. This has the effect of the prosthesis working in concert with the functional spine unit anatomy, thereby reducing nonphysiologic stresses and strains in the bony and soft tissue structures.

The benefits of a 3-component prosthesis, however, rely on the mobile core being truly mobile during the arc of motion. Laboratory and clinical studies of mobile core designs have shown that the core can get trapped due to stiction or poor positioning at the time of implantation. This can lead to stick-slip motion of the core, whereby the core is trapped and immobile over a portion of the FE motion of the spine and then released suddenly, resulting in high-velocity core motion, yielding a nonphysiologic kinematic signature characteristic of segmental instability.[39] This instability may result in increased muscle forces to control the instability as postulated by Panjabi.[41]

A mismatch between the lateral bending and axial rotation axes of the native segment and the prosthesis can cause abnormal facet contact and loading during these motions. Similarly, the uncinate processes may experience abutment because of abnormal motion coupling. During lateral bending, the cranial vertebra of the native segment undergoes a swinging motion within the bowl formed by the superior end plate and uncinate processes of the inferior vertebra. The axis of this swinging motion is in the cranial vertebral body. In contrast, a spherical bearing–implanted segment rotates about an axis of rotation in the caudal vertebral body, which is likely to result in abutment against the ipsilateral uncinate and increased tensile resistance of the soft tissue tether with the contralateral uncinate.[42] Such abnormal loading patterns in the facet joints and uncovertebral joints may lead to pain and further degeneration.

The design of a disc prosthesis can influence which anatomic components share the responsibility of resisting anterior shear motions and loads. An implanted segment may experience large shear forces depending on the sagittal alignment of the cervical spine and the orientation of the implanted segment relative to the gravitational load vector of the head acting through the external auditory meatus. A ball-and-socket articulation in a 2-component prosthesis bears the entire responsibility of resisting the shear forces that may act on the motion segment and transferring these shear stresses to the bone-prosthesis interface. On the other hand, a mobile core prosthesis that has no built-in resistance to shear allows the mobile core to translate until either the built-in stops become active, the facets engage or the soft tissues tension acts to block the shear motion at the implanted segment.

OTHER FACTORS

In addition to the prosthesis design features, several factors related to implantation of the prosthesis may influence the biomechanical response of cervical segments after disc arthroplasty. These factors include the amount of disc space distraction caused by the prosthesis height relative to the initial disc height; prosthesis placement in the sagittal and coronal planes; and integrity of the soft tissue envelope, which could be a balancing act between maintaining postoperative stability and releasing enough tissue to implant the prosthesis in what is considered optimal positioning for a given prosthesis design. A detailed discussion of how these factors influence the biomechanics of cervical segments after CDA is outside the scope of this article but can be found in a recent review article.[42]

SUMMARY

Meaningful differences between cervical disc prostheses come down to the allowed kinematic DOFs, location of the axis of rotation for a given motion, and device stiffness. How these device characteristics allow a prosthesis to work with the patient's anatomy, in the end, determines whether the prosthesis is successful at restoring motion and mitigating adjacent-level stresses. Biomechanical investigation has a strong role in defining these differences, but clinical data ultimately are needed to understand how individual prostheses function within a diseased or degenerative spine.

CLINICS CARE POINTS

- Prostheses that allow translation independent of rotation may better allow physiologic COR locations and, therefore, the physiologic loading of facets and the soft tissue envelope.
- A prosthesis with a compressible core may be best equipped to achieve the intended function of CDA and be more forgiving to placement errors.
- A disc prosthesis with built-in resistance to angular and translational motion can restore stability to a hypermobile segment without eliminating motion.
- Laboratory evidence suggests selection of a prosthesis design based on preoperative mobility of the index segment may result in improved motion quantity and quality.

DISCLOSURES AND CONFLICT OF INTEREST

A.G. Patwardhan: Consultant to Orthofix Medical Inc., Lewisville, TX, USA. Institutional research funds were received from Stryker (Kalamazoo, MI, USA), DePuy Synthes (Raynham, MA, USA), Orthofix Medical (Lewisville, TX, USA) and Medtronic (Memphis, TN, USA). R.M. Havey: Nothing to disclose.

REFERENCES

1. Robinson R, Smith G. Anterolateral cervical disc removal and interbody fusion for cervical disc syndrome. Bull John Hopkins Hosp 1955;96:223–4.
2. Bailey R, Badgely C. Stabilization of the cervical spine by anterior fusion. J Bone Joint Surg Am 1960;42:565–94.

3. Gore D, Sepic S. Anterior cervical fusion for degenerated or protruded discs: a review of one hundred forty-six patients. Spine 1984;9:667–71.

4. Bohlman H, Emery S, Goodfellow D, et al. Robinson anterior cervical discectomy and arthrodesis for cervical radiculopathy: long term follow-up of one hundred and twenty-two patients. J Bone Joint Surg Am 1993;75:1298–307.

5. Wigfield C, Gill S, Nelson R, et al. Influence of an artificial cervical joint compared with fusion on adjacent-level motion in the treatment of degenerative cervical disc disease. J Neurosurg 2002;96:17–21.

6. Bryan VE Jr. Cervical motion segment replacement. Eur Spine J 2002;11(suppl 2):S92–7.

7. McAfee PC, Cunningham B, Dmitriev A, et al. Cervical disc replacement-porous coated motion prosthesis: a comparative biomechanical analysis showing the key role of the posterior longitudinal ligament. Spine (Phila Pa 1976) 2003;28: S176–85.

8. Duggal N, Pickett GE, Mitsis DK, et al. Early clinical and biomechanical results following cervical arthroplasty. Neurosurg Focus 2004;17:E9.

9. Le H, Thongtrangan I, Kim DH. Historical review of cervical arthroplasty. Neurosurg Focus 2004;17:E1.

10. Pimenta L, McAfee PC, Cappuccino A, et al. Clinical experience with the new artificial cervical PCM (Cervitech) disc. Spine J 2004;4:315S–21S.

11. Traynelis VC. Cervical arthroplasty. Clin Neurosurg 2006;53:203–7.

12. Sasso RC, Smucker JD, Hacker RJ, et al. Artificial disc versus fusion: a prospective, randomized study with 2-year follow-up on 99 patients. Spine 2007; 32(26):2933–40.

13. Jaramillo-de la Torre JJ, Grauer JN, Yue JJ. Update on cervical disc arthroplasty: where are we and where are we going? Curr Rev Musculoskelet Med 2008;1:124–30.

14. Sasso R, Anderson P, Riew K, et al. Results of cervical arthroplasty compared with anterior discectomy and fusion: four-year clinical outcomes in a prospective, randomized, controlled trial. J Bone Joint Surg Am 2011;93:1684–92.

15. Coric D, Nunley PD, Guyer RD, et al. Prospective, randomized, multicenter study of cervical arthroplasty: 269 patients from the Kineflex C artificial disc investigational device exemption study with a minimum 2-year follow-up. J Neurosurg Spine 2011;15(4):348–58.

16. Zigler JE, Delamarter R, Murrey D, et al. ProDisc-C and anterior cervical discectomy and fusion as surgical treatment for single-level cervical symptomatic degenerative disc disease: five-year results of a Food and Drug Administration study. Spine 2013; 38(3):203–9.

17. Davis RJ, Kim KD, Hisey MS, et al. Cervical total disc replacement with the Mobi-C cervical artificial disc compared with anterior discectomy and fusion for treatment of 2-level symptomatic degenerative disc disease: a prospective, randomized, controlled multicenter clinical trial. J Neurosurg Spine 2013; 19(5):532–45.

18. Gornet MF, Burkus JK, Shaffrey ME, et al. Cervical disc arthroplasty with PRESTIGE LP disc versus anterior cervical discectomy and fusion: a prospective, multicenter investigational device exemption study. J Neurosurg Spine 2015;23(5):558–73.

19. Hisey MS, Zigler JE, Jackson R, et al. Prospective, randomized comparison of one-level Mobi-C cervical total disc replacement vs. anterior cervical discectomy and fusion: results at 5-year follow-up. Int J Spine Surg 2016;10:1–10. https://doi.org/10.14444/3010.

20. Sears W, McCombe P, Sasso R. Kinematics of cervical and lumbar total disc replacement. Semin Spine Surg 2006;18:117–29.

21. Büttner-Janz K. Classification of spine arthroplasty devices. In: Yu JJ, Bertagnoli R, McAfee PC, et al, editors. Motion preservation Surgery of the spine. Philadelphia, Pa, USA: Saunders Elsevier Press; 2008. p. 21–35.

22. Putzier M, Funk JF, Schneider SV, et al. Charité total disc replacement—clinical and radiographical results after an average follow-up of 17 years. Eur Spine J 2006;15(2):183–95.

23. Maislin G, Maislin DG, Keenan BT, et al. Preliminary Clinical Outcomes from the Polyetheretherketone on Ceramic Simplify™ Disc FDA IDE Trial. J Spine Neurosurg 2018;6:2.

24. Skeppholm M, Lindgren L, Henriques T, et al. The Discover artificial disc replacement versus fusion in cervical radiculopathy—a randomized controlled outcome trial with 2-year follow-up. The Spine J 2015;15(6):1284–94.

25. Finn MA, Brodke DS, Daubs M, et al. Local and global subaxial cervical spine biomechanics after single-level fusion or cervical arthroplasty. Eur Spine J 2009;18:1520–7.

26. Havey RM, Khayatzadeh S, Voronov LI, et al. Motion response of a polycrystalline diamond adaptive axis of rotation cervical total disc arthroplasty. Clin Biomech 2019;62:34–41.

27. Lauryssen C, Coric D, Dimmig T, et al. Cervical total disc replacement using a novel compressible prosthesis: Results from a prospective Food and Drug Administration–regulated feasibility study with 24-month follow-up. Int J Spine Surg 2012;6: 71–7.

28. Guyer RD, Voronov LI, Havey RM, et al. Kinematic assessment of an elastic-core cervical disc prosthesis in one and two-level constructs. JOR Spine 2018;1(4):e1040.

29. Lazennec JY, Aaron A, Ricart O, et al. The innovative viscoelastic CP ESP cervical disk prosthesis with six degrees of freedom: biomechanical concepts,

development program and preliminary clinical experience. Eur J Orthopaedic Surg Traumatol 2016; 26(1):9–19.

30. Patwardhan AG, Voronov L, Havey RM, et al. P152. Limited restoration of primary and coupled motions in lateral bending and axial rotation after total disc replacement: a common finding in cervical disc prostheses [abstract]. Spine J 2009;9(10): S192–3.

31. Puttlitz CM, Rousseau MA, Xu Z, et al. Intervertebral disc replacement maintains cervical spine kinetics. Spine (Phila Pa 1976) 2004;29:2809–14.

32. Puttlitz CM, DiAngelo DJ. Cervical spine arthroplasty biomechanics. Neurosurg Clin N Am 2005;16. 589–594, v.

33. Snyder JT, Tzermiadianos MN, Ghanayem AJ, et al. Effect of uncovertebral joint excision on the motion response of the cervical spine after total disc replacement. Spine (Phila Pa 1976) 2007;32:2965–9.

34. Patwardhan AG, Tzermiadianos MN, Tsitsopoulos PP, et al. Primary and coupled motions after cervical total disc replacement using a compressible six-degree-of-freedom prosthesis. Eur Spine J 2012;21(5):618–29.

35. Havey RM, Khayatzadeh S, Patwardhan AG. Thursday, September 27, 2018 3: 35 PM–5: 05 PM Section on Motion Technology Abstract Presentations: 135. Influence of preoperative segmental range of motion on postoperative motion after cervical disc arthroplasty using fixed-core, mobile-core and restrained compressible-core prostheses. The Spine J 2018;18(8):S66–7.

36. Patwardhan AG, Havey RM, Khayatzadeh, S. Influence of prosthesis design on the relationship between preoperative and postoperative flexion-extension ROM after cervical disc arthroplasty. Presented at the Global Spine Congress, May 15–18, 2019, Toronto, Canada.

37. Martin S, Ghanayem AJ, Tzermiadianos MN, et al. Kinematics of cervical total disc replacement adjacent to a two-level, straight versus lordotic fusion. Spine 2011;36(17):1359–66.

38. Lee MJ, Dumonski M, Phillips FM, et al. Disc replacement adjacent to cervical fusion: a biomechanical comparison of hybrid construct versus two-level fusion. Spine 2011;36(23):1932–9.

39. Patwardhan AG, Havey RM. Prosthesis design influences segmental contribution to total cervical motion after cervical disc arthroplasty. Eur Spine J 2019;1–9.

40. Milne N. The role of zygapophysial joint orientation and uncinate processes in controlling motion in the cervical spine. J Anat 1991;178:189.

41. Panjabi MM. The stabilizing system of the spine. Part II. Neutral zone and instability hypothesis. J Spinal Disord 1992;5:390–6. discussion 397.

42. Patwardhan AG, Havey RM. Biomechanics of Cervical Disc Arthroplasty—A Review of Concepts and Current Technology. Int J Spine Surg 2020;14(s2): S14–28.

Adjacent-Segment Disease Following Spinal Arthroplasty

Jonathan M. Parish, MD[a],*, Anthony M. Asher, BA[b], Domagoj Coric, MD[c,d]

KEYWORDS

- Cervical disc replacement • Lumbar disc replacement • Arthroplasty • Adjacent level disease
- Motion preservation

KEY POINTS

- Spinal arthroplasty preserves motion and reduces adjacent segment stress.
- Adjacent segment disease is a multifactorial process.
- The annual incidence of adjacent segment disease following fusion is relatively low (1%–2%); therefore, early studies with low patient numbers and/or short-term follow-up were not powered sufficiently to show significant differences in arthroplasty and arthrodesis.
- Long-term studies indicate that arthroplasty may result in fewer adjacent segment reoperations.

INTRODUCTION

Adjacent segment (AS) degeneration and disease have been contentious topics for decades, virtually since the introduction of spinal arthrodesis. The advent of spinal arthroplasty has only served to intensify since this controversy. AS degeneration is defined as new degenerative radiographic changes at a spinal level immediately above or below surgically treated levels. When this degeneration is associated with clinical symptoms such as radiculopathy, myelopathy, or mechanical instability, it is deemed AS disease. AS disease, requiring reoperation, more objectively defines clinically significant AS disease. The development of AS disease is multifactorial, including factors such as natural progression of the underlying degenerative process or patient-specific factors (eg, global alignment, bone density), as well as increased biomechanical stress placed on ASs following fusion surgery. Theoretically, motion-preserving devices should mitigate any accelerated degeneration related to fusion and increased

biomechanical stress. AS disease is a difficult entity to empirically study because of inherently low rates of AS reoperation after fusion. Therefore, large patient series/meta-analyses and/or long-term follow-up are needed to demonstrate significant differences between fusion and arthroplasty. As more studies comparing spinal arthrodesis to arthroplasty with long-term follow-up become available for review and meta-analysis, there is growing evidence basis to support the concept that arthroplasty positively affects the incidence of AS disease and reoperation.

HISTORICAL PERSPECTIVE

Historically, the annual incidence of AS disease (clinical symptoms) following fusion is widely variable, but is generally reported to range from 1% to 5%.[1–4] Hilibrand's[4] seminal article reported 409 total anterior cervical fusion procedures in 374 patients with 10-year follow-up. In this series, symptomatic AS disease was defined, in a non-standardized fashion, as a combination of new

---

[a] Department of Neurological Surgery, Carolinas Medical Center, 1000 Blythe Boulevard, Charlotte, NC 28203, USA; [b] University of North Carolina School of Medicine, 1000 Blythe Boulevard, Charlotte, NC 28203, USA; [c] Carolina Neurosurgery and Spine Associates, 225 Baldwin Avenue, Charlotte, NC 28204, USA; [d] Atrium Musculoskeletal Institute, Charlotte, NC, USA
* Corresponding author.
E-mail address: John.parish@cnsa.com

Neurosurg Clin N Am 32 (2021) 505–510
https://doi.org/10.1016/j.nec.2021.05.009
1042-3680/21/© 2021 Elsevier Inc. All rights reserved.

radicular or myelopathic symptoms referrable to a level adjacent to the index cervical fusion on 2 consecutive office visits based on retrospective chart review and surgical records. The annual incidence of AS disease using these nonvalidated criteria was reported as 2.9% per year over the 10-year study period. However, only 27 patients (6.6%) had AS reoperation, with an annual AS reoperation rate of 0.66%. The study by Goffin and colleagues[5] is another frequently cited large retrospective study looking at incidence of AS disease following anterior cervical fusion (ACDF). These investigators evaluated long-term outcomes in 180 patients with radiographic and clinical follow-up greater than 60 months (mean 100.9 months). Nearly all patients (92%) had AS degeneration (radiographic changes) at long-term follow-up, whereas only 6.1% underwent AS reoperation (0.7% per year). This rate is remarkably similar to the AS reoperation rate reported by Hilibrand.

EARLY ARTHROPLASTY STUDIES AND ADJACENT SEGMENT DISEASE

Some early cervical arthroplasty studies with short-term follow-up (<4 years) and/or limited number of patients suggested no or small differences in AS disease between fusion and arthroplasty, fueling some controversy concerning the effect of motion preservation on ASs. This controversy is not surprising though, given the inherently low rate of AS reoperation, as noted by Hilibrand and Goffin.[4,5] A meta-analysis of single-level arthroplasty versus fusion failed to show significant clinical difference in AS disease at 24 months.[6] Although AS disease was only addressed in a single study that was included in the meta-analysis, the investigators concluded "total disc arthroplasty does not affect the incidence of adjacent segment disease." Similarly, Jawahar and colleagues[7] reported 93 patients in 3 separate Food and Drug Administration (FDA) IDE trials for 1- and 2-level cervical arthroplasty. They found equivalent neurologic outcomes with no significant difference in AS disease (15% for ACDF vs 18% for total disc replacement [TDR]). The investigators did not discuss adjacent level reoperation; instead, they defined AS disease as radiographic changes with clinical symptoms requiring an active intervention. Despite the relatively small number of patients and only short-term follow-up, the investigators concluded that arthroplasty fails to reduce the risk of developing AS disease. More recently, this same author group (Utter and colleagues[8]) reported a statistically significant reduction ($P = .0001$) in AS reoperation of TDR (4.3%) versus ACDF (14.8%) at 7-year follow-up, supporting the need for large patient series and/or long-term follow-up in order to demonstrate significant differences in AS disease. A more recent randomized study[9] with a relatively small number of patients (ACDF = 34, TDR = 32) and only short-term follow-up (2 years) concluded, "Adjacent segment degeneration parameters were comparable...." A single institution study by Coric and colleagues[10] included 2 TDR devices with a total of 63 patients and 4-year follow-up. Both arthroplasty and ACDF patients showed a low rate of AS reoperation (4.9% vs 3.0%, respectively) without a statistically significant difference. Although these are well-designed randomized studies, the small patient numbers and short term (<4 year follow-up) limit the interpretation of the potential effect on AS disease and reoperation.

Other early studies with larger patient numbers showed more promising potential effects of motion preservation on AS disease. In 2013, Davis and colleagues[11] reported the results of the Mobi-C IDE study, demonstrating statistically significant lower AS disease after 2 level arthroplasty versus ACDF at 24-month follow-up ($P = .03$). Six patients (5.7%) required revision with extension of fusion after ACDF versus 2 patients (0.9%) after TDR at 24 months. Robertson and colleagues[12] reported 74 patients after ACDF and 154 patients after Bryan Disc TDR (Medtronic Sofamor Danek, Inc). After 24 months, AS disease was significantly higher after fusion ($P = .018$).

ADJACENT SEGMENT REOPERATION

Studies addressing AS reoperation rate provide the most objective assessment of the clinical effect of motion preservation on adjacent levels. This criterion (AS reoperation) is objective, a simple binary yes or no, and, inarguably clinically meaningful. In a single-institution study by Coric and colleagues,[13] lower AS reoperation rates were observed for arthroplasty than fusion. Ninety patients were randomized to ACDF (37 patients) or cervical disc arthroplasty (53 patients) with 2-year minimum follow-up (mean 38 months). AS reoperation occurred at a rate of 1.7% (0.5% per year) in the arthroplasty group compared with 8.1% (2.6% per year) in the ACDF group, although this did not reach statistical significance likely because of the relatively low patient numbers. The same author (Coric[14]) reported the results of the multicenter, prospective, randomized Kineflex-C (Spinal Motion, Inc) Investigational Device Exemption (IDE) study, which addressed AS degeneration (radiographic) as well as AS reoperation rates. A total of 269 patients were enrolled with 135 patients randomized to TDR and 133 to fusion. At 2-year follow-up, severe AS degeneration was evident in 24.8% of ACDF patients and only 9% in TDR group (P<.0001). There was no significant difference in AS reoperation rate (7.6% for TDR and 6.1% for fusion), again, likely because of the short-term follow-up. Burkus and colleagues[15] reported the results of the multicenter, prospective, randomized Prestige Disc ST (Medtronic, Inc) IDE study of 541 patients. They demonstrated a rate of AS reoperation of 2.9% after TDR versus 4.9% after ACDF (P = .376) at minimum follow-up of 24 months, not reaching statistical significance. However, the same investigators[16] reported the same cohort with long-term follow-up (7-year) and reported AS reoperation rates statistically significantly less for the arthroplasty group (4.6% vs 11.9%, P = .008). Upadhyaya and colleagues[17] published a meta-analysis that included full data from 3 randomized, multicenter, FDA IDE studies (Prestige ST, Bryan, and ProDisc-C [Centinel Spine, LLC]). A total of 621 patients received an artificial disc, and 592 patients were treated with cervical fusion. At 24 months, the rate of secondary surgery at the index level was significantly lower for arthroplasty with a relative risk (RR) of 0.44 (95% confidence interval [CI], 0.26–0.77, P = .004, I^2 = 0%). There was also a significant reduction in the AS reoperation risk favoring arthroplasty with an RR of 0.460 (95% CI, 0.229–0.926, P = .030, I^2 = 2.9%). These trends suggested a benefit of motion preservation on AS disease.

Given the low incidence of AS reoperation following fusion (~1%), long-term studies and a large number of patients are required to adequately assess the potential positive effect of motion preservation and to show statistically significant differences. Vaccaro and colleagues[18] reported the results of the prospective, multicenter, randomized FDA Secure-C (Globus Medical) IDE trial. At 2 years, patients in the TDR group had a nonstatistically significant lower rate of AS reoperation compared with ACDF (1.7% vs 3.5, respectively) Subsequently, this difference was reported as statistically significant at 7-year follow-up (TDR = 3.8% vs ACDF = 13.2%).[19] Phillips and colleagues[20] also reported 7-year outcomes from the PCM artificial disc (NuVasive, Inc) IDE study with significantly less AS disease after arthroplasty and lower rate of secondary surgeries (index or adjacent level) (8.5% vs 13.0%). These prospective, randomized, long-term follow-up studies have provided firm evidence basis for the benefit of motion preservation on AS reoperations.

Long-term results after 2-level cervical disc arthroplasty have also shown a positive effect

on adjacent level operations. Radcliff and colleagues[21] reported 5-year results from the Mobi-C (Zimmer-Biomet) IDE study of 330 patients undergoing 2-level TDR versus ACDF. There were statistically significantly fewer AS reoperations in TDR group than in the ACDF group (3.1% vs 11.4%, P = .0004). For TDR, the annual rate of AS reoperation was 0.6% per year, which is slightly lower than the actual reoperation rate (0.66% per year) reported by Hilibrand. There were also statistically significantly fewer second surgeries at the index level in the TDR group compared with the ACDF group (7.1% vs 21.0%, P = .0006). Furthermore, the investigators also reported AS degeneration with TDR showing significantly less AS degeneration (50.7% vs 90.5%, P<.0001). Notably, the rate of AS radiographic degeneration in this ACDF cohort was almost identical to the rate reported in Goffin's[5] earlier ACDF study. Recently, Lanman and colleagues[22] reported the results of the 2-level IDE study for the Prestige LP (Medtronic, Inc) TDR at 7-year follow-up, which showed less AS reoperation for TDR (6.5%) versus ACDF (12.5%).

Radcliff and colleagues[23] reported a retrospective, matched cohort analysis of patients enrolled in a Blue Cross Plan treated with TDR or ACDF. There were a total of 6635 patients in the ACDF group and 327 patients in the cervical TDR group. At 36 months, the incidence of AS reoperation was significantly lower for TDR group compared with the ACDF group (5.7% vs 10.5%, respectively). The patients in this study were not part of IDE trials and therefore were thought to represent "real-world" outcomes, supporting a lower incidence AS reoperation following arthroplasty.

LUMBAR ARTHROPLASTY

Although first described in the 1960s by Fernström,[24] there is a relative paucity of research on AS disease in lumbar TDR. The first FDA-approved device, SB Charité III Artificial Disc (DePuy Spine Inc), was cleared for clinical use in the United States in 2004. Currently, there are only 2 FDA-approved lumbar TDR devices available for use in the United States, ProDisc-L (Centinel) and activL (Aesculap, Inc). There was significant early excitement concerning the potential of lumbar arthroplasty to reduce AS stress given the relatively high rate of reoperation (up to 15% at 10 years) after lumbar fusion in long-term studies.[25,26] Although some studies addressing AS disease and AS reoperation have suggested that there may be a lower rate of AS disease following lumbar arthroplasty, others simply demonstrate clinical noninferiority of TDR compared with fusion.

Lumbar Adjacent Segment Disease and Reoperation

Multiple long-term case series of different devices have shown low rates of AS disease requiring AS reoperation after lumbar arthroplasty. Aghayev and colleagues[27] published a 5-year analysis of large series with 248 patients enrolled in the SWISS Spine Registry, a nationwide registry for lumbar TDA. At 5-year follow-up, 10.7% of patients had AS degeneration (radiographic), all in the cranially AS, and no patients in the study underwent AS reoperation. A smaller single-site series by Lu and colleagues[28] reported 30 patients undergoing lumbar TDR with the SB Charité III Artificial Disc with long-term mean follow-up of 15.2 years. Over this long-term follow-up, 19 patients (63.3%) developed radiologic AS degeneration, although only 1 patient (3.3%) underwent AS reoperation. Lazennec and colleagues[29] published a 5-year follow-up of 61 patients who underwent lumbar TDR with LP-ESP (FH Orthopedics) implant. No patients underwent surgery for AS disease in the 5-year follow-up period, and all patients maintained AS disc height within 25% of normal. In 2018, Plais and colleagues[30] published an analysis of 87 patients who underwent lumbar TDR with the Maverick TDR (Medtronic, Inc), 61 of whom had a 10-year follow-up. Nearly half (42.5%) of the patients underwent a hybrid procedure with an anterior lumbar interbody fusion at 1 level and a TDR at an adjacent level. At 10-year follow-up, 12.9% of patients were deemed to have AS degeneration, which the investigators defined as 50% decrease in disc space height. Only 3 patients (4.8% or 0.5% per year) underwent AS reoperation. The investigators concluded that arthroplasty did not protect against AS disease but also did not accelerate AS disease. Although overall patient numbers are relatively low in most of these series, the incidence of AS reoperation appears low following lumbar TDR with long-term follow-up.

Long-Term Comparison with Lumbar Fusion

Long-term comparative studies of fusion versus lumbar arthroplasty provide additional insight into the effect of motion preservation on AS disease. Rainey and colleagues[31] conducted a large retrospective study in 2012, reviewing 1000 patients who underwent lumbar TDR along with 67 patients who underwent lumbar fusion. Rates of AS reoperation were higher in the fusion cohort (4.5%) than in the TDR cohort (2.0%) at a mean length to reoperation of 28.3 months (range, 0.5–85 months), although this was not statistically significant. Furthermore, 30% of the patients in the TDR cohort who required AS reoperation had preexisting severe degeneration at the adjacent level, and the investigators suggest that the rate of AS reoperation after arthroplasty may be lower if appropriate patients/levels were addressed. Two large, randomized trials have also addressed long-term AS disease following arthroplasty and fusion. Zigler and colleagues[32] randomized patients to 236 patients to single-level arthroplasty with ProDisc-L (Centinel) or circumferential fusion. At 5-year follow-up, AS degeneration (radiographic) was observed in 9.2% of arthroplasty patients and 28.6% of fusion patients ($P = .004$), and AS reoperation was reported in 1.9% of TDR patients and 4.0% of fusion patients ($P = .689$). New AS degeneration, that is, preoperatively no adjacent level disease, was reported in 6.7% of TDR patients and 23.8% of fusion patients ($P = .008$). In 2018, Radcliff and colleagues[33] published a randomized controlled trial involving 229 patients who underwent either 2-level circumferential fusion or 2-level TDR for degenerative disk disease between L3 and S1. They found that the TDR group underwent significantly lower secondary surgeries in the 5-year postoperative period (5.6% vs 19.1%, $P = .0027$). The secondary surgeries occurred at the index level 65% of the time, and there was no significant difference in the rates of reoperation for AS disease between the 2 cohorts, although rates trended lower after TDR (2.5% vs 5.9%, $P = .24$). These studies indicate a positive effect of arthroplasty on AS disease but were not powered properly to detect a statistically significant difference between arthroplasty and fusion.

Two meta-analyses have been performed addressing AS disease following lumbar TDR. A meta-analysis[34] of 926 fusion patients and 313 TDR patients in 19 studies evaluated AS degeneration. Thirty-four percent of fusion patients and 9% of TDR patients developed AS degeneration ($P<.0001$). In regard to AS disease, 16 studies were included with 1216 fusion patients and 595 TDR patients. Symptomatic AS disease occurred in 14% of fusion patients and 1% of TDR patients ($P<.0001$). A second, more recent, meta-analysis[35] with a total of 13 studies addressing AS disease and reoperation included 1270 patients. The prevalence of AS disease was significantly higher after fusion ($P = .0008$ and $P<.0001$, respectively), and this prevalence was apparent in both short-term (<5 years) and long-term (>5 years) follow-up.

SUMMARY

AS degeneration (radiographic) and AS disease (clinical) are multifactorial processes that include modifiable factors, such as surgical technique and choice of surgical procedure (eg, arthroplasty vs arthrodesis), as well as nonmodifiable factors, such as natural history of the underlying degenerative disease. AS disease is most objectively and relevantly quantified by the rate of AS reoperation, which appears to be relatively low (∼1–2% per year) following fusion. Therefore, any meaningful attempt to assess the effect of motion-preserving devices on AS reoperation requires large patient numbers or long-term (5-year or greater) follow-up. Reports with relatively small patient numbers and short term (2 years or less) are not appropriately powered to detect statistically significant differences. Studies with long-term follow-up have provided a growing body of evidence to suggest that TDR positively effects the incidence of AS disease.

CLINICS CARE POINTS

- Arthroplasty in the cervical and lumbar spine has shown a trend toward less adjacent segment degeneration.
- Arthroplasty in the cervical and lumbar spine has also shown a positive trend of fewer adjacent segment reoperations in long-term studies.

CONFLICT-OF-INTEREST DISCLOSURES (D. CORIC):

- Globus Medical: Consultant/Royalties
- Spine Wave: Consultant/Stock/Royalties
- Medtronic: Consultant/Royalties
- Stryker Spine: Consultant/Royalties
- RTI Surgical: Royalties
- Integrity Implants: Consultant/Royalties
- Premia Spine: Consultant/Stock
- United Healthcare: Spine Advisory Board.

REFERENCES

1. Bohlman HH, Emery SE, Goodfellow DB, et al. Robinson anterior cervical discectomy and arthrodesis for cervical radiculopathy. Long-term follow-up of one hundred and twenty-two patients. J Bone Joint Surg Am 1993;75(9):1298–307.
2. Cauthen JC, Kinard RE, Vogler JB, et al. Outcome analysis of noninstrumented anterior cervical discectomy and interbody fusion in 348 patients. Spine 1998;23(2):188–92.
3. Gore DR, Sepic SB. Anterior discectomy and fusion for painful cervical disc disease. A report of 50 patients with an average follow-up of 21 years. Spine 1998;23(19):2047–51.
4. Hilibrand AS, Carlson GD, Palumbo MA, et al. Radiculopathy and myelopathy at segments adjacent to the site of a previous anterior cervical arthrodesis. J Bone Joint Surg Am 1999;81(4):519–28.
5. Goffin J, Geusens E, Vantomme N, et al. Long-term follow-up after interbody fusion of the cervical spine. J Spinal Disord Tech 2004;17(2):79–85.
6. Bartels RHMA, Donk R, Verbeek ALM. No justification for cervical disk prostheses in clinical practice: a meta-analysis of randomized controlled trials. Neurosurgery 2010;66(6):1153–60 [discussion 1160].
7. Jawahar A, Cavanaugh DA, Kerr EJ, et al. Total disc arthroplasty does not affect the incidence of adjacent segment degeneration in cervical spine: results of 93 patients in three prospective randomized clinical trials. Spine J 2010;10(12):1043–8.
8. Utter A, Nunley PD, Kerr EJ, et al. Risk of clinical adjacent segment pathology risk through 7 years postop is reduced following cervical disc arthroplasty compared to ACDF. J Neurosurg Spine 2019;30(3):1–135.
9. Vleggeert-Lankamp CLA, Janssen TMH, van Zwet E, et al. The NECK trial: effectiveness of anterior cervical discectomy with or without interbody fusion and arthroplasty in the treatment of cervical disc herniation; a double-blinded randomized controlled trial. Spine J 2019;19(6):965–75.
10. Coric D, Kim PK, Clemente JD, et al. Prospective randomized study of cervical arthroplasty and anterior cervical discectomy and fusion with long-term follow-up: results in 74 patients from a single site. J Neurosurg Spine 2013;18(1):36–42.
11. Davis RJ, Kim KD, Hisey MS, et al. Cervical total disc replacement with the Mobi-C cervical artificial disc compared with anterior discectomy and fusion for treatment of 2-level symptomatic degenerative disc disease: a prospective, randomized, controlled multicenter clinical trial: clinical article. J Neurosurg Spine 2013;19(5):532–45.
12. Robertson JT, Papadopoulos SM, Traynelis VC. Assessment of adjacent-segment disease in patients treated with cervical fusion or arthroplasty: a prospective 2-year study. J Neurosurg Spine 2005; 3(6):417–23.
13. Coric D, Cassis J, Carew JD, et al. Prospective study of cervical arthroplasty in 98 patients involved in 1 of 3 separate investigational device exemption studies from a single investigational site with a minimum 2-year follow-up. Clinical article. J Neurosurg Spine 2010;13(6):715–21.
14. Coric D, Nunley PD, Guyer RD, et al. Prospective, randomized, multicenter study of cervical arthroplasty: 269 patients from the Kineflex C artificial disc investigational device exemption study with a

minimum 2-year follow-up: clinical article. J Neurosurg Spine 2011;15(4):348–58.

15. Kenneth Burkus J, Haid RW, Traynelis VC, et al. Long-term clinical and radiographic outcomes of cervical disc replacement with the prestige disc: results from a prospective randomized controlled clinical trial: presented at the 2009 Joint Spine Section Meeting. J Neurosurg Spine 2010;13(3):308–18.

16. Burkus JK, Tranelis VC, Hiad RW, et al. Clinical and radiographic analysis of an artifical cerical disc: 7-year follow-up from the Prestige prospective randomized controlled clinical trial: Clinical article. J Neurosurg Spine 2014;21(4):516–28.

17. Upadhyaya CD, Wu J-C, Trost G, et al. Analysis of the three United States Food and Drug Administration investigational device exemption cervical arthroplasty trials. J Neurosurg Spine 2012;16(3):216–28.

18. Vaccaro A, Beutler W, Peppelman W, et al. Clinical outcomes with selectively constrained SECURE-C cervical disc arthroplasty: two-year results from a prospective, randomized, controlled, multicenter investigational device exemption study. Spine 2013;38(26):2227–39.

19. Vaccaro A, Beutler W, Peppelman W, et al. Long-term clinical experience with selectively constrained SECURE-C cervical artificial disc for 1-level cervical disc disease: results from seven-year follow-up of a prospective, randomized, controlled investigational device exemption clinical trial. Int J Spine Surg 2018;12(3):377–87.

20. Phillips FM, Geisler FH, Gilder KM, et al. Long-term outcomes of the US FDA IDE prospective, randomized controlled clinical trial comparing PCM cervical disc arthroplasty with anterior cervical discectomy and fusion. Spine 2015;40(10):674–83.

21. Radcliff K, Coric D, Albert T. Five-year clinical results of cervical total disc replacement compared with anterior discectomy and fusion for treatment of 2-level symptomatic degenerative disc disease: a prospective, randomized, controlled, multicenter investigational device exemption clinical trial. J Neurosurg Spine 2016;25(2):213–24.

22. Lanman TH, Burkus JK, Dryer RG, et al. Long-term clinical and radiographic outcomes of the Prestige LP artificial cervical disc replacement at 2 levels: results from a prospective randomized controlled clinical trial. J Neurosurg Spine 2017;27(1):7–19.

23. Radcliff K, Zigler J, Zigler J. Costs of cervical disc replacement versus anterior cervical discectomy and fusion for treatment of single-level cervical disc disease: an analysis of the Blue Health Intelligence database for acute and long-term costs and complications. Spine 2015;40(8):521–9.

24. Fernström U. Arthroplasty with intercorporal endoprothesis in herniated disc and in painful disc. Acta Chir Scand Suppl 1966;357:154–9.

25. Okuda S, Nagamoto Y, Matsumoto T, et al. Adjacent segment disease after single segment posterior lumbar interbody fusion for degenerative spondylolisthesis: minimum 10 years follow-up. Spine 2018; 43(23):E1384–8.

26. Nakashima H, Kawakami N, Tsuji T, et al. Adjacent segment disease after posterior lumbar interbody fusion: based on cases with a minimum of 10 years of follow-up. Spine 2015;40(14):E831–41.

27. Aghayev E, Etter C, Bärlocher C, et al. Five-year results of lumbar disc prostheses in the SWISSspine registry. Eur Spine J 2014;23(10):2114–26.

28. Lu S, Sun S, Kong C, et al. Long-term clinical results following Charite III lumbar total disc replacement. Spine J 2018;18(6):917–25.

29. Lazennec J-Y, Rakover J-P, Rousseau M-A. Five-year follow-up of clinical and radiological outcomes of LP-ESP elastomeric lumbar total disc replacement in active patients. Spine J 2019;19(2):218–24.

30. Plais N, Thevenot X, Cogniet A, et al. Maverick total disc arthroplasty performs well at 10 years follow-up: a prospective study with HRQL and balance analysis. Eur Spine J 2018;27(3):720–7.

31. Rainey S, Blumenthal SL, Zigler JE, et al. Analysis of adjacent segment reoperation after lumbar total disc replacement. Int J Spine Surg 2012;6:140–4.

32. Zigler JE, Glenn J, Delamarter RB. Five-year adjacent-level degenerative changes in patients with single-level disease treated using lumbar total disc replacement with ProDisc-L versus circumferential fusion: clinical article. J Neurosurg Spine 2012;17(6):504–11.

33. Radcliff K, Spivak J, Darden B 2nd, et al. Five-year reoperation rates of 2-level lumbar total disk replacement versus fusion: results of a prospective, randomized clinical trial. Clin Spine Surg 2018;31(1): 37–42.

34. Harrop JS, Youssef JA, Maltenfort M, et al. Lumbar adjacent segment degeneration and disease after arthrodesis and total disc arthroplasty. Spine 2008; 33(15):1701–7.

35. Ren C, Song Y, Liu L, et al. Adjacent segment degeneration and disease after lumbar fusion compared with motion-preserving procedures: a meta-analysis. Eur J Orthop Surg Traumatol 2014; 24(Suppl 1):S245–53.

Lumbar Total Disc Replacement: Current Usage

Daniel Franco, MD*, Garrett Largoza, BA, Thiago S. Montenegro, MD,
Glenn A. Gonzalez, MD, Kevin Hines, MD, James Harrop, MD, MSHQS

KEYWORDS

- Lumbar disc replacement • Total disc arthroplasty • Artificial disc

KEY POINTS

- Lumbar disc replacement technologies have made considerable advancements since they initially came to market.
- Careful patient selection is paramount to ensure success. Motion preservation technologies are not a universal solution.
- LDR offers similar results than anterior-posterior fusion but has significantly shorter operative time, less blood loss and shorter recovery period.

INTRODUCTION

Low back pain is the leading cause of disability worldwide in industrial nations.[1,2] The pathology underlying chronic low back pain is associated with numerous factors including aging, mechanical overloading, and genetic factors. Lumbar degenerative disc disease, which refers to the gradual depreciation, desiccation, and loss of function of intervertebral discs, is a major source of low back pain.[3]

There are several treatment modalities that can be employed for patients with low back pain. Nonsurgical treatment options for degenerative disc disease exist in the form of pain management through a combination of anti-inflammatory medications and steroid injections, physical therapy that focuses on strengthening the postural lumbar musculature, and lifestyle modifications.[4] Studies have shown that surgical intervention is more effective in relieving low back pain caused by segmental motion or instability in patients with severe unremitting chronic symptoms.[5–7] Surgical intervention historically employed spinal fusion surgery, which in essence unites adjacent vertebrae. Spinal fusion or arthrodesis eliminates the natural motion between vertebrae and potentially can have negative impacts on the surrounding structures because of creation of alterative loading mechanisms. Some potential adverse developments include new adjacent degenerative changes resulting in radiculopathies and new or worsened low back pain.[5] Lumbar spinal fusion surgery decreases focal segmental mobility, leading to increased mechanical stress on the neighboring vertebrae, which can further accelerate degeneration within the lumbar spine.[6,7] This phenomenon is referred to adjacent level disease. To avoid potential negative effects of arthrodesis in addition to preserving maximal range of motion of the lumbar spine, lumbar disc replacement surgery has been adopted as an alternative to fusion treatment for severe, chronic low back pain and degenerative disc disease.

One of the first primitive iterations of lumbar disc replacement (LDR) came from Fernström in the 1960s.[8] He surgically placed stainless steel balls in the disc spaces in the cervical and lumbar spine. He reportedly achieved similar results to fusion in the short term, but his implants were plagued with significant complications as a result of subsidence and extrusions. Only a couple of decades later, at the Charité Hospital in Germany, the first modern disc replacement implant (Charité I) was designed.

Department of Neurological Surgery, Thomas Jefferson University Hospitals, 909 Walnut Street, Room 320L, Philadelphia, PA 19107, USA
* Corresponding author.
E-mail address: daniel.franco@jefferson.edu

Neurosurg Clin N Am 32 (2021) 511–519
https://doi.org/10.1016/j.nec.2021.05.010
1042-3680/21/© 2021 Elsevier Inc. All rights reserved.

Total lumbar disc replacement was introduced first in the United States in 2004, with US Food and Drug Administration (FDA) approval of the Charité disc prosthesis from Depuy Synthes (**Fig. 1**). The Charite device was later removed from the market in 2012. Shortly after entrance of the Charite device, Prodisc-L from Centinel Spine was subsequently approved by the FDA, in 2006 (**Fig. 2**). After a 10-year hiatus, Activ-L from Aesculap (**Fig. 3**) was brought to market in 2015. Presently, the Prodisc –L and Activ-L are available for patient usage in the United States. These devices now serve as an effective alternative to spinal fusion. Their design provides for relative preservation of segmental load transfer and stability with greater reduction in back pain and disability in patients who undergo total disc replacement surgery compared with those who receive spinal fusion surgery or nonsurgical intervention based on randomized clinical studies.[9,10]

CURRENT LUMBAR DISC REPLACEMENT OPTIONS

Lumbar total disc replacement (LDR) is an alternative to arthrodesis with the potential benefit of preserving spinal motion of the intervertebral segment and avoiding extra loading at adjacent levels.[11] Since the approval of LDR by the FDA in 2004, it has been shown to be effective in numerous prospective clinical trials. These results have illustrated that LDR is an option for symptomatic single-and 2-level lumbar degenerative disc disease in a select patient population.[12–17] Numerous spine societies, including international organizations (North American Spine Society [NASS], National Institute for Health and Care Excellence [NICE], Health Care Quality Ontario [HQO], Europe, Medical & Scientific Advisory Committee [MSAC], and International Society for the Advancement of Spine Surgery [ISASS]), have published recommendations supporting LDR utilization for patients and recommended coverage by payors based on reliable tools, validated clinical outcomes, and long-term safety data.[12,18–23]

Industry has introduced several artificial discs and noted differences, similarities, and specificities in their constructs over other devices. However, there are 3 main biomechanical properties of a natural disc that are aimed to be reproduced:

1. Toleration of load without failure
2. Reduction of bony friction and wear
3. Conservation of range of motion (ROM)[24]

Lumbar artificial disc devices can be classified according to their composition and regarding to

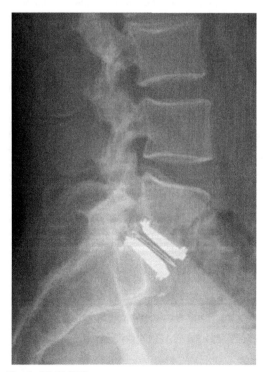

Fig. 1. L5-S1 LDR.

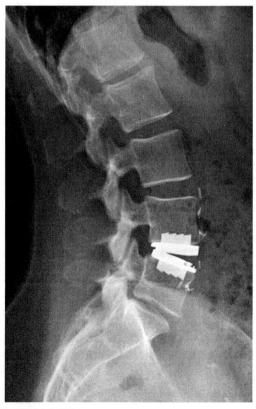

Fig. 2. L4-5 LDR.

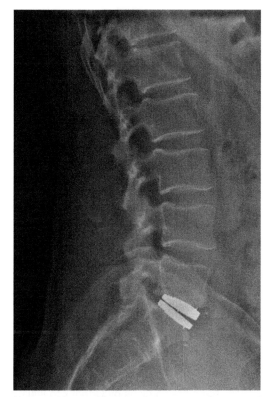

Fig. 3. L5-S1 LDR with ActivL. © B. Braun Melsungen AG.

their limitation to the ROM of the device. Articulating discs are composed of 2 or 3 solid components combined in a ball-in-socket display and can be considered to have a constrained or semiconstrained design; Maverick, ProDisc, and ActivL are examples of this type of device. This design provides for a more physiologic range of motion but at the expense of shock absorption, as they do not have a compressive component present in other designs. Nonarticulating disc devices are more complex structures with a soft core, and have unconstrained designs providing for 6 degrees of freedom segmental motion; Charité is an example of this device.[5,24,25] The literature describes that constrained prostheses with a limited curvature cause increased facet joint wear and tear in extension, and on the other hand unconstrained implants that translate during extension may be able to find an equilibrium between facet load and capsuloligamentous tension.[26]

Different disc cores presently available on the market consist of either ultrahigh molecular weight polyethylene (UHMWPE) or polycarbonate urethane (PCU). UHMWPE is a stiffer material, inert and more resistant to delamination with a smoother self-lubricating surface that gives it a lower risk of wear and tear, making it ideal in high-friction zones and allowing it to serve better

as a joint. These particular properties made UHMWPE popular in the manufacturing of knee and hip replacement prosthetics. Most of the first artificial discs launched used this technology, like Charite, and ProDisc L.[5,27,28] Despite the fact that UHMWPE plays an important role in imitating a natural joint surface, its stiffness makes it unfavorable to shock absorption from repetitive loads. Newer polymers seem to have improved biomechanical material and like PCU are now being used in the core of new-generation nonarticulating implants like the M6 (Orthofix, Lewisville, Texas), a popular implant choice in Europe.[29]

The following sections describe arthroplasty devices and manufactures that have been available in the market for a lumbar total disc replacement.

SB Charité (DePuy Spine, Raynham, Massachusetts)

Charité I, developed in 1982 at the Charité Hospital in Berlin, was the first artificial disc used in the lumbar spine in 1984. Specifically, it consisted of 2 highly polished metal endplates and an UHMWPE sliding core articulating between these endplates.[30,31] It was subsequently modified in 1985 to the second version because of axial migration and in some cases even disarticulation. This SB Charité II had metal endplates enlarged with anchoring teeth to improve the support to the metallic endplates of the vertebral body. The Charité III design used up until its removal from market was first produced in 1987. Changes and improvement were required in the Charité II after fractures in the endplates and insufficient instrumentation for implantation. Charité III changed the endplates cast to a Cobalt-Chromium-Molybdenum (CoCrMo) alloy, and introduced new angulated endplates of 5°, 7.5°, and 10° that can be combined with each other to improve lordotic reconstruction of the lumbar spine. Later, a porous coating of the endplates was introduced to promote osteointegration, but the main design basically remained unchanged until the device was discontinued from the market in 2012.[5,24,31]

ProDisc artificial total lumbar disc replacement (Centinel Spine, West Chester, Pennsylvania)

Similar to Charité, ProDisc I was developed in the 1980s first by Aesculpa then Depuy/Sythesis Spine. This device is considered a composite artificial disc, comprised of several articulating parts of different materials, and also used a polymeric UHMWPE core and metallic endplates. However, different from Charité, it has only a single articulating interface between the polyethylene core fixed to the superior and inferior metallic end plate, and it has a semiconstrained articulated design.[5,24,32,33] After some refinements, in 1999 ProDisc II was launched. and has been used since FDA approval in 2006, currently being manufactured by Centinel Spine.

MAVERICK artificial disc (Medtronic Sofamor Danek, Incorporated, Memphis, Tennessee)

The first metal-on-metal artificial disc design, made of articulating parts made of a single type of material, was the Maverick disc, conceived in 2002. The articulating parts were made out of a cobalt-chromium alloy in a semiconstrained design with increased height compared with other models and a fixed center of rotation, resulting in the facets being partially unloaded.[5,26,32] The US FDA IDE trial for the device was completed, but it has never received FDA approval, despite long-term follow-up data from the IDE trial group in the United States[13] and Europe[34] showing that the device is safe and effective in treating single-level lumbar degenerative disc disease.

FlexiCore (Stryker, Incorporated, Kalamazoo, Michigan) and Kineflex (Spinal Motion, Incorporated, Montain View, California)

These are both lumbar arthroplasty devices with a fixed center of rotation; however, Flexicore has a fully constrained design, while Kineflex/L is composed of metal endplates with a mobile core positioned between 2 base plates, giving it a semiconstrained design.[26,32] Both artificial discs completed the US FDA IDE trial, but neither was submitted for or received FDA approval.

Recently Launched Devices

Activ-L (Aesculap, Incorporated, Center Valley, Pennsylvania)

Activ-L is a next-generation metal polymer-metal articulating disc, which gives the device a mobile center of rotation; it was approved by the FDA in 2015. It has a semiconstrained design with 3 modular components, inferior and superior cobalt-chrome-molybdenum (CoCrMo) plates, and similar to ProDisc-L, an UHMWPE inlay lying inside the inferior plate[32,35] (**Fig. 4**).

M6-L (Orthofix, Incorporated, Lewisville, Texas)

M6-L incorporated PCU in its core to add a shock absorbance capacity and a limited ROM. It is a 1-piece device and has an elastomeric design; in other words, the core is designed to adapt and deform as a natural disc would, imitating both the nucleus pulposus and the outer annulus properties. It is not FDA approved for lumbar disc replacement; however, its version for cervical spine was recently FDA approved in 2019. Currently there are no plans by Orthofix to initiate an FDA submission or US clinical trial for approval of the M6-L. Initial European data show that this design is safe and durable.[36] However, more long-term studies have to be done before a definitive assessment can be made.

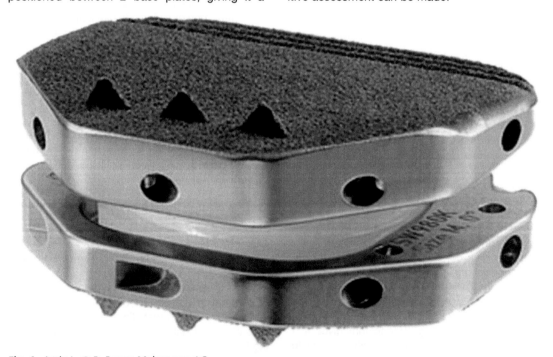

Fig. 4. Activ-L. © B. Braun Melsungen AG.

CURRENT TRENDS OF USE FOR LUMBAR DISC REPLACEMENT

Currently in the United States, Prodisc-L and Activ-L are the only FDA-approved implants that remain on the market. There is compelling, level 1 evidence and subsequent long-term outcomes data that these devices offer a different and effective approach to the treatment of degenerative disc disease (DDD) with a similar complication profile than traditional fusion techniques.[14,37,38] An important advantage of these implants over fusion is the potential for reduction of adjacent-level degeneration when patients are selected appropriately.[37,39] LDR has been in use in Europe since the mid-1980s, and the results from the European experience have been favorable, even in long-term follow-up of 7 to 10 years.[38,40] Despite all this, LDR is still trying to get traction in the North American market; the hold of spinal fusion in the US market remains very strong, in part influenced by both reduced compensation and a higher rate of insurance denial compared with similar spinal fusion procedures.

A study published by Yoshihara found that the surgical treatment for lumbar DDD increased 2.4-fold in the United States from 2000 to 2009, with a decrease in LDR and an increase in fusion procedures in the same time period.[41] Other authors analyzed the Nationwide Inpatient Sample (NIS) database from 2000 to 2008 and found similar results. Steady growth in lumbar spinal fusion was reported, with a 28% decrease in the number of lumbar arthroplasty procedures.[42] On the same vein, a study published by Saifi and colleagues[43] found that from 2005 to 2013, primary LDR significantly declined in the United States by 86%, notwithstanding several studies guiding to enhanced efficacy and cost-efficiency.

Recent studies analyzed these trends and found that the reduction in the LDR use was associated with poor surgical indications, adverse events with off-label use, lack of support from the insurance companies, and technical challenges.[42] This inequality may be associated with a reduction of surgeon compensation from insurance companies. Congruently, the number of revision LDR cases has decreased 30%, while the revision burden for spinal fusions has risen from 6% to 24%.[43]

INDICATIONS AND CONTRAINDICATIONS FOR LUMBAR DISC REPLACEMENT

Lumbar arthroplasty was designed to restore the physiologic movement of a healthy intervertebral disc and prevent excessive loading of the adjacent levels.[11] Based on the FDA IDE study inclusion and exclusion criteria,[14,44] the ideal candidate for LDR is a patient with discogenic or mechanical low back pain without evidence of radiculopathy or structural compromise (ie, spondylolisthesis or fractures). Wong and colleagues[45] also added that patients considered to be good candidates for LDR are typically earlier in the Kirkaldy-Willis[46] degenerative cascade than a fusion patient. Generally, LDR is considered only after the patient has failed more than 6 months of nonoperative therapies. LDR can be performed for various indications currently, including patients with prior microdiscectomy and those with prior fusions with adjacent segment disease.[44,47,48] Similar to the workup before a fusion procedure, the data needed to make the determination of recommending LDR to a patient include history, pain and disability scores, clinical and imaging findings (flexion-extension radiographs, computed tomography [CT] and magnetic resonance imaging [MRI] scans), prior diagnostic procedures as well as support systems (family or friends).

As mentioned before, the body of literature describes a very specific and ideal candidate for LDR, all based on the clinical trials and follow-up long-term data. On the other hand, there are a significant number of contraindications, albeit mostly relative, that prevent a more wide-spread use of LDR technologies. Büttner-Janz and colleagues[49] described them best in their 2014 article, divided into 7 main groups:

1. General: active infection or malignancy, renal failure and/or active hepatitis, osteomyelitis, neuromuscular disease, ankylosed spine, pregnancy, psychosocial disorders
2. Anatomic: pars fracture, spondylolisthesis, compression fracture, disc collapse with < 3-4 mm disc space, facet ankylosis and degeneration, history of laminectomy, scoliosis, irregular endplate shape, pseudoarthrosis
3. Subsidence risk: osteoporosis, endocrine and metabolic disorders (hyperparathyroidism, Cushing syndrome), Paget disease, chronic steroid use
4. Pathology: radiculopathy, arachnoiditis, stenosis, multilevel operation needed (beyond 1–2 levels), previous spine surgery at the affected level (except for microdiscectomy without facet violation), fibromyalgia
5. Implant rejection: history of hypersensitivity to protein pharmaceuticals or collagen, history of implant rejection, metal allergy, anaphylaxis
6. Approach related: obesity, aberrant vascular anatomy, major vascular calcification, previous abdominal and vascular surgeries, prior

retroperitoneal radiation, prior surgery at the affected level

7. Other: previous exposure to any or all bone morphogenic proteins

COMPLICATIONS AFTER LUMBAR DISC REPLACEMENT

The reported complications profile following total lumbar disc arthroplasty is similar to that of an anterior lumbar interbody fusion (ALIF); a significant portion of these are actually not dependent on the implant itself but rather on the anterior retroperitoneal approach that is required in order to reach the lower lumbar levels.[50] The first iteration of Charité, being one of the oldest implants, has the greatest number of reported adverse events in the literature.[50] In 1 retrospective review series,[51] both early and late complications were detailed. Early complications, defined as occurring within the first year after implantation, included prosthesis axial dislocation, abdominal hematoma, retrograde ejaculation, subsidence, and infection. Late complications were more often related to the biomechanics and design of the implant, such as prosthesis subsidence and migration, adjacent level degeneration, facet arthrosis at the level of the implant, and polyethylene wear of the implant with subsequent collapse of the implanted level.[48,49] From an economics perspective, although LDRs do have a higher revision rate (11.2% vs 5.8% respectively) than a similar AP fusion, the cost of these are offset by the significantly shorter length of stay and overall lower hospital costs,[52] which makes these implants an attractive option for health systems to carry in their portfolio of services.

Holt[50] clarified in 2007 that a key point lost in the literature is that most complications that occur after LDR are unrelated to a specific device but more likely because of a technique. Vascular injury is a relatively common problem while preforming an anterior approach to the lumbar spine; this is further complicated when implanting disc replacement device, as these often require precise insertion in the midline, as well as wide exposure of the disc space, which in turn means that large vessels have to be aggressively retracted and manipulated. Subsidence can occur in a small subset of LDRs; some authors argue that this may be in part due to an issue with proper technique.[53] Consider that while it is important to perform a complete disc removal and endplate preparation, removal of the outer cortex of the endplate will expose soft cancellous bone that is unable to support the prosthesis. Sizing the implant appropriately is also paramount; ideally the device should

cover as much of the outer vertebral cortical bone as possible, providing the strongest possible foundation for the implant to sit. Other technique-related complications include excessive facet distraction, pedicle fracture, vertebral body split fractures (especially in devices with a keel), development of scoliotic deformities, and spontaneous fusion caused by malposition implants.[26]

Management of complications following LDR can be a daunting and challenging task. There are limited data in the literature analyzing the different strategies that can be used. In general terms, excluding all perioperative- and approach-related complications (vessel injury, retrograde ejaculation) after a failed LDR spine surgeons tend to favor definitive revision surgery and conversion into a circumferential fusion. Some of the more experienced LDR surgeons will, however, consider removing the faulty implant and replacing it with a new one, especially if the patient had responded well symptomatically, and imaging showed no overt degeneration of the level of interest or adjacent structures.[38,54] Some authors also argue that in cases of mechanical pain without new neurologic dysfunction and with preserved implant integrity, the addition of posterior pedicle screw fixation can be enough to immobilize a segment with a previous LDR[55] and improve the patient's symptoms. In all, when performing revision surgery for LDR, one needs to have a reliable and experienced access surgeon, take great care and consideration of surrounding vascular structures, and be very methodical and deliberate when removing the faulty implant; if considering reimplantation with another LDR device, careful inspection of endplate structure and integrity is also necessary.

SUMMARY

The LDR has been shown to be a safe and effective alternative to lumbar fusions. Zigler and Delamarter[44] published extensive follow-up data on the early iterations of LDR; they showed that most patients maintained improvement of Oswestry-Disability Scores, even 5 years after implant placement, and there were significantly fewer cases of adjacent segment disease compared with similar lumbar fusions.[54,56] The economics seem to favor LDR also; multiple authors have concluded that overall patients undergoing LDR as opposed to a circumferential fusion spend less time in the operating room with shorter anesthesia time, have a smaller blood loss, and have shorter hospitalizations.[57,58] Following this trend, in May 2020, the FDA approved the use of Prodisc-L (Centinel Spine) for up to 2-level LDR, illustrating the growing confidence of the market in this surgical solution; studies that led to this approval demonstrated that multilevel lumbar disc arthroplasty is an alternative to arthrodesis and offers clinical advantages in terms of pain relief and functional recovery.[59] An in vitro cadaveric study in the military compared 2-level arthroplasties versus similar circumferential fusions and found that the latter significantly increased load and biomechanical strain in the adjacent facet joints, whereas the 2-level arthroplasties preserved most natural physiologic range of motion.[60] Long-term follow-up studies support the use of multilevel arthroplasty in patients with significant disc degeneration without major facet arthropathies or central canal stenosis. The data in these suggests that there is much better preservation of the natural range of motion of the spine, not only on the affected levels that are receiving the implant but also of the cranial and caudal adjacent levels, even as far as 6 years down the line.[48,61]

LDRs have been undergone constant reinvention and improvement over the last few decades, and the latest designs offer safe and effective preservation of motion. There are questions regarding the durability and lifelong consequences of this devices that remain to be answered, but the experience from current implants appears promising.[26] The current literature available shows that with judicious patient selection and when set indication criteria are met, lumbar disc arthroplasty can be a powerful tool in a spine surgeon's armamentarium.

DISCLOSURE

The authors have nothing to disclose.

REFERENCES

1. GBD 2017 Disease and Injury Incidence and Prevalence Collaborators. Global, regional, and national incidence, prevalence, and years lived with disability for 354 diseases and injuries for 195 countries and territories, 1990-2017: a systematic analysis for the Global Burden of Disease Study 2017. Lancet 2018;392:1789–858.
2. Andersson GB. Epidemiological features of chronic low-back pain. Lancet 1999;354:581–5.
3. Manchikanti L, Singh V, Falco FJ, et al. Epidemiology of low back pain in adults. Neuromodulation 2014; 17(Suppl 2):3–10.
4. Battié MC, Joshi AB, Gibbons LE. Degenerative disc disease: what is in a name? Spine (Phila Pa 1976) 2019;44:1523–9.
5. Othman YA, Verma R, Qureshi SA. Artificial disc replacement in spine surgery. Ann Transl Med 2019;7:S170.
6. Bai D-y, Liang L, Zhang B-B. Total disc replacement versus fusion for lumbar degenerative diseases-a meta-analysis of randomized controlled trials. Medicine (Baltimore) 2019;98:e16460.
7. Johnstone B, Bayliss MT. The large proteoglycans of the human intervertebral disc. Changes in their biosynthesis and structure with age, topography, and pathology. Spine (Phila Pa 1976) 1995;20:674–84.
8. Fernström U. Arthroplasty with intercorporal endoprothesis in herniated disc and in painful disc. Acta Chir Scand Suppl 1966;357:154–9.
9. Kos N, Gradisnik L, Velnar T. A brief review of the degenerative intervertebral disc disease. Med Arch 2019;73:421–4.
10. Yajun W, Yue Z, Xiuxin H, et al. A meta-analysis of artificial total disc replacement versus fusion for lumbar degenerative disc disease. Eur Spine J 2010;19: 1250–61.
11. McAfee PC. The indications for lumbar and cervical disc replacement. Spine J 2004;4:S177–81.
12. Gornet M, Buttermann G, Guyer R, et al. Defining the ideal lumbar total disc replacement patient and standard of care. Spine (Phila Pa 1976) 2017;42: S103–7.
13. Gornet M, Burkus J, Dryer R, et al. Lumbar disc arthroplasty versus anterior lumbar interbody fusion: five-year outcomes for patients in the Maverick disc IDE study. New Orleans (LA): Spine Arthroplasty Society; 2010.
14. Guyer RD, McAfee PC, Banco RJ, et al. Prospective, randomized, multicenter Food and Drug Administration investigational device exemption study of lumbar total disc replacement with the CHARITE artificial disc versus lumbar fusion: five-year follow-up. Spine J 2009;9:374–86.
15. Sköld C, Tropp H, Berg S. Five-year follow-up of total disc replacement compared to fusion: a randomized controlled trial. Eur Spine J 2013;22:2288–95.
16. Chung SS, Lee CS, Kang CS. Lumbar total disc replacement using ProDisc II: a prospective study with a 2-year minimum follow-up. Clin Spine Surg 2006;19:411–5.
17. Park S-J, Lee C-S, Chung S-S, et al. Long-term outcomes following lumbar total disc replacement using ProDisc-II: average 10-year follow-up at a single institute. Spine (Phila Pa 1976) 2016;41:971–7.
18. NASS. NASS coverage policy recommendations: lumbar artificial disc replacement. 2019. Available at: https://www.spine.org/coverage.
19. NICE. National Institute for Health and Care Excellence. Prosthetic intervertebral disc replacement in the lumbar spine. Interventional procedures guidance.2019. Available at: https://www.nice.org.uk/guidance/ipg306.

20. Medical Advisory Secretariat. Artificial discs for lumbar and cervical degenerative disc disease–update: an evidence-based analysis. Ont Health Technol Assess Ser 2006;6:1.

21. Aesculap. Reimbursement of lumbar TDR devices, Europe. 2018. Available at: https://www.aesculapimplantsystems.com/en/patients/about-your-lumbar-spine/disc-replacement-surgery/reimbursement-information.htm.

22. MSAC M. Review of interim funded service: artificial intervertebral disc replacement lumbar 2011. p. 170. Report I ed: MSAC Available at: http://www.msac.gov.au/internet/msac/publishing.nsf/Content/5DE3C448FF252171CA25801000123B66/$File/1090.1-Assessment-Report.pdf.

23. Zigler J, Garcia R. ISASS policy statement–lumbar artificial disc. Int J Spine Surg 2015;9.

24. Salzmann SN, Plais N, Shue J, et al. Lumbar disc replacement surgery—successes and obstacles to widespread adoption. Curr Rev Musculoskelet Med 2017;10:153–9.

25. Choi J, Shin D-A, Kim S. Biomechanical effects of the geometry of ball-and-socket artificial disc on lumbar spine: a finite element study. Spine (Phila Pa 1976) 2017;42:E332–9.

26. Sandhu FA, Dowlati E, Garica R. Lumbar arthroplasty: past, present, and future. Neurosurgery 2020;86:155–69.

27. Veruva SY, Lanman TH, Isaza JE, et al. Periprosthetic UHMWPE wear debris induces inflammation, vascularization, and innervation after total disc replacement in the lumbar spine. Clin Orthop Relat Res 2017;475:1369–81.

28. Veruva SY, Steinbeck MJ, Toth J, et al. Which design and biomaterial factors affect clinical wear performance of total disc replacements? A systematic review. Clin Orthop Relat Res 2014;472:3759–69.

29. St John KR. The use of compliant layer prosthetic components in orthopedic joint repair and replacement: a review. J Biomed Mater Res B Appl Biomater 2014;102:1332–41.

30. Putzier M, Funk JF, Schneider SV, et al. Charité total disc replacement—clinical and radiographical results after an average follow-up of 17 years. Eur Spine J 2006;15:183–95.

31. Link HD. In: History, design and biomechanics of the LINK SB Charite artificial disc. Arthroplasty of the spine. Springer; 2004. p. 36–43.

32. Palepu V, Kodigudla M, Goel VK. Biomechanics of disc degeneration. Adv Orthop 2012;2012:726210.

33. Beatty S. We need to talk about lumbar total disc replacement. Int J Spine Surg 2018;12:201–40.

34. Assaker R, Ritter-Lang K, Vardon D, et al. Maverick total disc replacement in a real-world patient population: a prospective, multicentre, observational study. Eur Spine J 2017;26:1417.

35. Sun W, Wang P, Hu H, et al. Retrospective study on effectiveness of Activ L total disc replacement. J Orthop Surg Res 2021;16:1–7.

36. Schätz C, Ritter-Lang K, Gössel L, et al. Comparison of single-level and multiple-level outcomes of total disc arthroplasty: 24-month results. Int J Spine Surg 2015;9:14.

37. Rainey S, Blumenthal SL, Zigler JE, et al. Analysis of adjacent segment reoperation after lumbar total disc replacement. Int J Spine Surg 2012;6:140–4.

38. Zigler JE, Sachs BL, Rashbaum RF, et al. Two- to 3-year follow-up of ProDisc-L: results from a prospective randomized trial of arthroplasty versus fusion. SAS J 2007;1:63–7.

39. Zigler JE, Blumenthal SL, Guyer RD, et al. Progression of adjacent-level degeneration after lumbar total disc replacement: results of a post-hoc analysis of patients with available radiographs from a prospective study with 5-year follow-up. Spine (Phila Pa 1976) 2018;43:1395–400.

40. Tropiano P, Huang RC, Girardi FP, et al. Lumbar total disc replacement. Seven to eleven-year follow-up. J Bone Joint Surg Am 2005;87:490–6.

41. Yoshihara H, Yoneoka D. National trends in the surgical treatment for lumbar degenerative disc disease: United States, 2000 to 2009. Spine J 2015;15:265–71.

42. Awe OO, Maltenfort MG, Prasad S, et al. Impact of total disc arthroplasty on the surgical management of lumbar degenerative disc disease: analysis of the nationwide inpatient sample from 2000 to 2008. Surg Neurol Int 2011;2:139.

43. Saifi C, Cazzulino A, Park C, et al. National trends for primary and revision lumbar disc arthroplasty throughout the United States. Glob Spine J 2018;8:172–7.

44. Zigler JE, Delamarter RB. Five-year results of the prospective, randomized, multicenter, Food and Drug Administration investigational device exemption study of the ProDisc-L total disc replacement versus circumferential arthrodesis for the treatment of single-level degenerative disc disease. J Neurosurg Spine 2012;17:493–501.

45. Wong DA, Annesser B, Birney T, et al. Incidence of contraindications to total disc arthroplasty: a retrospective review of 100 consecutive fusion patients with a specific analysis of facet arthrosis. Spine J 2007;7:5–11.

46. Kirkaldy-Willis WH, Wedge JH, Yong-Hing K, et al. Pathology and pathogenesis of lumbar spondylosis and stenosis. Spine (Phila Pa 1976) 1978;3:319–28.

47. Mayer HM, Wiechert K, Korge A, et al. Minimally invasive total disc replacement: surgical technique and preliminary clinical results. Eur Spine J 2002;11(Suppl 2):S124–30.

48. Bertagnoli R, Yue JJ, Shah RV, et al. The treatment of disabling multilevel lumbar discogenic low back pain with total disc arthroplasty utilizing the ProDisc

prosthesis: a prospective study with 2-year minimum follow-up. Spine (Phila Pa 1976) 2005;30:2192–9.

49. Büttner-Janz K, Guyer RD, Ohnmeiss DD. Indications for lumbar total disc replacement: selecting the right patient with the right indication for the right total disc. Int J Spine Surg 2014;8:12.

50. Holt RT, Majd ME, Isaza JE, et al. Complications of lumbar artificial disc replacement compared to fusion: results from the prospective, randomized, multicenter US Food and Drug Administration investigational device exemption study of the Charité artificial disc. SAS J 2007;1:20–7.

51. van Ooij A, Oner FC, Verbout AJ. Complications of artificial disc replacement: a report of 27 patients with the SB Charité disc. J Spinal Disord Tech 2003;16:369–83.

52. Kurtz SM, Lau E, Ianuzzi A, et al. National revision burden for lumbar total disc replacement in the United States: epidemiologic and economic perspectives. Spine (Phila Pa 1976) 2010;35:690–6.

53. McAfee PC, Geisler FH, Saiedy SS, et al. Revisability of the Charite artificial disc replacement: analysis of 688 patients enrolled in the U.S. IDE study of the Charite artificial disc. Spine (Phila Pa 1976) 2006;31:1217–26.

54. Zigler JE, Glenn J, Delamarter RB. Five-year adjacent-level degenerative changes in patients with single-level disease treated using lumbar total disc replacement with ProDisc-L versus circumferential fusion. J Neurosurg Spine 2012;17:504–11.

55. Cunningham BW, Hu N, Beatson HJ, et al. Revision strategies for single- and two-level total disc arthroplasty procedures: a biomechanical perspective. Spine J 2009;9:735–43.

56. Stubig T, Ahmed M, Ghasemi A, et al. Total disc replacement versus anterior-posterior interbody fusion in the lumbar spine and lumbosacral junction: a cost analysis. Glob Spine J 2018;8:129–36.

57. Siepe CJ, Heider F, Wiechert K, et al. Mid- to long-term results of total lumbar disc replacement: a prospective analysis with 5- to 10-year follow-up. Spine J 2014;14:1417–31.

58. Levin DA, Bendo JA, Quirno M, et al. Comparative charge analysis of one- and two-level lumbar total disc arthroplasty versus circumferential lumbar fusion. Spine (Phila Pa 1976) 2007;32:2905–9.

59. Delamarter R, Zigler JE, Balderston RA, et al. Prospective, randomized, multicenter Food and Drug Administration investigational device exemption study of the ProDisc-L total disc replacement compared with circumferential arthrodesis for the treatment of two-level lumbar degenerative disc disease: results at twenty-four months. J Bone Joint Surg Am 2011;93:705–15.

60. Dmitriev AE, Gill NW, Kuklo TR, et al. Effect of multilevel lumbar disc arthroplasty on the operative- and adjacent-level kinematics and intradiscal pressures: an in vitro human cadaveric assessment. Spine J 2008;8:918–25.

61. Rasouli A, Cuellar JM, Kanim L, et al. Multiple-level lumbar total disk replacement: a prospective clinical and radiographic analysis of motion preservation at 24-72 months. Clin Spine Surg 2019;32:38–42.

Posterior Lumbar Facet Replacement and Arthroplasty

Ben Jiahe Gu, MD, Rachel Blue, MD*, Jang Yoon, MD,
William C. Welch, MD, FICS

KEYWORDS

● Facet replacement ● Arthroplasty ● Degenerative spine disease ● Motion preservation

KEY POINTS

● Motion-preserving facet replacement devices have been shown to preserve near-normal spinal motion while providing stability in ex vivo models.
● Clinical trials so far have demonstrated similar outcomes between facet arthroplasty and traditional fusion for lumbar spinal stenosis.
● It remains to be seen whether facet arthroplasty improves clinical outcomes with regard to symptoms and the development of adjacent segment disease.

INTRODUCTION
Nature of the Problem

Lumbar degenerative spine disease, encompassing conditions such as spondylolisthesis, disc degeneration, and lumbar spinal stenosis, has been estimated to have a global incidence of 3.63%.[1] Patients with degenerative disease of the lumbar spine frequently suffer from symptoms such as lower back pain, lower extremity pain, and lower extremity weakness, which significantly diminish their quality of life. While symptomatic control can often be achieved with nonsurgical treatments, many patients benefit from surgical intervention.[2,3] Instrumented fusion is widely performed to address spinal instability in lumbar degenerative spine disease,[4] which is traditionally implicated in the pathophysiology of axial mechanical back pain.[5,6] Pedicle screw-rod construct has been the workhorse of modern spinal stabilization technique to achieve rigid fixation until the bone growth occurs across the fusion surface.

However, rigid fixation technique may result in mixed clinical results in treating the symptoms of lumbar degenerative spine disease,[7] and while instrumentation enhances fusion rate, it does not necessarily correlate with improved clinical outcome.[8] To explain these discrepancies, it has been hypothesized that abnormal load distribution across vertebral endplates may play a major role in mechanical back pain and is not optimally addressed by spinal fusion, which can produce a normal loading pattern but may lead to sagittal imbalance, placing abnormal loads on adjacent segments.[9] Indeed, a major complication of spinal fusion is adjacent segment degeneration secondary to biomechanical alterations, which can eventually lead to clinical deterioration and reoperation.[10]

Seeking to address shortcomings of rigid fixation and solid fusion, various motion preservation devices have been introduced for the treatment of lumbar degenerative spine disease. While the exact mechanisms of these devices remain poorly defined, most are designed to limit spinal motion without causing abnormal load-bearing and associated degeneration of adjacent segments.[9] In the following sections, the authors present the

Disclosure: The authors have no financial conflicts of interest to disclose.
Department of Neurosurgery, Perelman School of Medicine, University of Pennsylvania, 3rd Floor, Silverstein Pavilion, 3400 Spruce Street, Philadelphia, PA 19104, USA
* Corresponding author.
E-mail address: Rachel.Blue@pennmedicine.upenn.edu

Neurosurg Clin N Am 32 (2021) 521–526
https://doi.org/10.1016/j.nec.2021.05.011
1042-3680/21/© 2021 Elsevier Inc. All rights reserved.

categories of these motion preservation devices and hone in on facet replacement devices, the primary focus of this review.

Definitions

"Motion preservation devices" in the context of treating lumbar degenerative spine disease can be broadly categorized into prosthetic devices and dynamic stabilization devices (**Fig. 1**). Prosthetic devices such as total disc, nucleus, and facet replacement devices aim to replace structures in the lumbar motion segment. In contrast, dynamic stabilization devices such as posterior dynamic stabilization devices (PDS) and interspinous process distraction devices work to control motion and load bearing of the index segments without replacing any anatomic structures. In this review, the authors discuss prosthetic devices for facet replacement and arthroplasty.

Goals of Facet Replacement and Arthroplasty

In cases of severe facet tropism, facet hypertrophy, facet arthropathy, and spinal stenosis, partial or full laminectomy with facetectomy can be used to relieve patients of low back and leg pain. While patients often attain good relief of neurologic symptoms with decompression alone, various clinical class II studies have shown that decompression with fusion improves outcomes related to axial mechanical back pain.[11,12] Accordingly, decompression combined with fusion is the gold standard of treatment, but as previously discussed, rigid fixation and solid fusion is associated with loss of spinal motion and adjacent segment degeneration. Facet arthroplasty serves as an alternative to spinal fusion after decompression and aims to stabilize the spine while preserving normal intervertebral motion of the index segments. It allows for wide decompression, laminectomy, and bilateral total facetectomy. In the following section, the authors discuss the various devices that have been developed for lumbar facet replacement and arthroplasty.

DISCUSSION
Considerations

In general, a motion-preserving facet replacement device must possess several key characteristics. It must be firmly secured to the cephalad and caudal spinal levels. This is especially important because unlike traditional hardware for rigid fixation, which only needs to persist until completion of bony fusion, the facet replacement device must maintain its integrity indefinitely. Moreover, while the attachment points must be rigid, they must be connected in a fashion that allows for mobility so that motion of the spine can be preserved. This mobility must mimic the biomechanics of native facet joints to maintain physiologic load distribution and range of motion for the index and adjacent segments. Thus, it is crucial to study candidate devices preclinically for its biomechanical properties. Finally, general considerations such as biocompatibility and durability must be stressed as with any joint replacement implant. In the following sections, the authors present the three existing facet

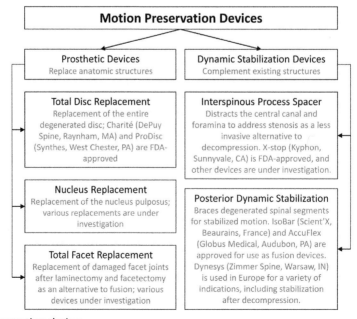

Fig. 1. Motion preservation devices.

replacement devices with a discussion of how they address these requirements. Each discussion will encompass device design, preclinical studies, and clinical experience.

Anatomic Facet Replacement System

The Anatomic Facet Replacement System (AFRS; Facet Solutions Inc, Logan, Utah) was designed based on a computed tomographic morphology study of the facet joint.[13] The system uses traditional titanium pedicle screw fixation to secure its superior and inferior facet implants, which are connected via cross-linking members to provide stability. The implant is made from a cobalt-chromium-molybdenum alloy, which has been successfully used in other metal total joint replacement systems.[14,15] The backing of the implant that interfaces with bone is treated with titanium plasma spray and hydroxyapatite coating to promote bony in-growth.

In terms of preclinical evidence, AFRS was validated in an in vitro study using cadaveric osteoligamentous segments (L3-S1).[16] After destabilization via L4-L5 complete bilateral facetectomy, it was shown that AFRS can restore range of motion and intradiscal pressure under physiologic loads to approximate intact spine. Importantly, screw-to-bone interface stress with AFRS was found to be minimal, indicating the potential for lasting hardware stability.

Regarding clinical experience, the United States Food and Drug Administration granted an Investigational Device Exemption (IDE) approval in 2006 to conduct a clinical trial for AFRS in the treatment of lumbar spinal stenosis. A Pivotal Study of a Facet Replacement System to Treat Spinal Stenosis (NCT00401518) enrolled 390 patients and was completed in 2017. While full results have not been published, preliminary outcomes at two and 4 years postoperatively for 213 randomized patients demonstrated comparable improvements in mean Zurich Claudication Questionnaire (ZCQ) and visual analog scale (VAS) scores between treatment (patients receiving AFRS) and control (patients receiving instrumented posterolateral fusion) arms.[17] Mean operative time was greater for the treatment arm (148 vs 126 minutes), as was estimated blood loss (381 vs 344 mL). Rates of subsequent surgery at the index level were comparable between groups. Together, these results suggest that AFRS may be a safe and effective treatment of lumbar spinal stenosis as an alternative to instrumented posterolateral fusion.

However, a 2018 case report described development of cobalt allergy, local tissue reaction, and return of neurologic symptoms after a pain-free interval (<2 years) in 2 of 5 patients receiving the implant at one institution.[18] Both patients required implant removal and revision to instrumented fusion, which were uncomplicated. These cases raise the concern that metal-on-metal facet replacement devices such as AFRS can release fine debris that lead to immune reaction and subsequent implant failure.

Total Facet Arthroplasty System

The Total Facet Arthroplasty System (TFAS; Archus Orthopedics, Inc, Redmond, Wash) consists of cephalad "L"-shaped stems secured to a caudal bearing system that allows for motion. The bearing system resembles a sphere sliding along a curved plate. The construct is anchored via pegs passing into the vertebral body along the same course as traditional pedicle screws and is secured using polymethyl methacrylate bone cement. It is composed of implantation-grade metal and is offered in a range of sizes to accommodate specific anatomy of each patient.

Preclinically, TFAS was well studied for its biomechanical properties. In human cadaveric lumbar spine models, TFAS was shown to restore stability while allowing near-normal spinal motion after wide decompressive laminectomy and bilateral facetectomy at L3-4,[19] L4-L5,[20] and L5-S1.[21] Moreover, unlike rigid fixation, it was shown to restore normal disc pressures after L4-L5 decompression, suggesting restoration of anterior column load-sharing.[22] Together, these results suggested that TFAS can stabilize the lumbar spine after wide decompression while maintaining near-physiologic range of motion and load distribution.

Compared with AFRS described previously and the Total Posterior Arthroplasty System (TOPS), which will be discussed in the next section, relatively little clinical experience exists for the application of TFAS. In a prospective observational study, 13 patients with degenerative spinal stenosis received TFAS implant at L3-L4 or L4-L5 after decompressive laminectomy and inferior facet resection and were followed up for an average of 3.7 years.[23] All patients demonstrated improvement on VAS and Oswestry Disability Index (ODI) without significant complications. Four patients demonstrated radiographic progression of their degeneration at index and adjacent levels but no clinical deterioration.

A phase 3 randomized controlled multicenter IDE clinical trial (NCT00418197), TFAS Clinical Trial, which sought to compare TFAS to posterior fusion, was discontinued for financial reasons, and interim results were never published.

However, a single-center case report described stem breakage at 9 and 27 months postoperatively in two patients who received total facet replacement at L4-L5 for grade 1 spondylolisthesis with stenosis. Both patients received uncomplicated salvage transpsoas instrumented fusion, as a posterior approach was suboptimal because of the presence of bone cement in the vertebral body, increasing the risk of pseudoarthrosis, and an anterior approach was limited by obesity. The authors of this report hypothesized that repetitive caudocephalad loading of pedicle screws led to fatigue and breakage.[24]

Total Posterior Arthroplasty System

The TOPS (Premia Spine, Ltd, Philadelphia, Pa) is an unitary device consisting of titanium plates connected by a polycarbonate urethane (PcU) articulating core. The plates have protrusion arms that are secured to cephalad and caudal vertebrae with pedicle screws, which are coated with hydroxyapatite to promote bony ingrowth. The PcU core provides limited range of motion to the construct but also absorbs shock, decreasing load transfer to adjacent spinal levels and to the implant-bone interface, lowering risk of construct failure. Moreover, it covers articulating surfaces, preventing release of possible debris from wear.

In vitro, TOPS was implanted and tested in fresh cadaveric lumbar segments to study its biomechanical properties.[25] In this study, TOPS preserved normal motion after laminectomy and bilateral facetectomy. It reduced intradiscal pressure but still allowed the disc to participate in load sharing. Adjacent segment motion was not significantly altered by TOPS implantation. Finally, it was shown that, compared with the Dynesys system (Zimmer Biomet, Warsaw, Ind), a PDS device with 6% to 8% screw loosening rate at 2 to 3 years postoperatively, load transmission to the TOPS pedicle screws is 36% less at the screw-bone interface during flexion and extension and 46% less during lateral bending. Together, these results suggest that TOPS can provide stabilization, preserve motion, and retain its integrity as an alternative to rigid fixation and solid fusion after decompressive laminectomy and total facetectomy.

In terms of clinical experience, a multicenter prospective pilot study of 29 patients with spinal stenosis and/or spondylolisthesis at L4-5 due to facet arthropathy received laminectomy and bilateral total facetectomy followed by TOPS implantation.[25] Patients were followed up to 1 year, and outcomes on VAS, ODI, and ZCQ improved significantly over the follow-up period. Radiographic studies demonstrated no further degeneration, no hardware malfunction, and preserved global spinal motion of flexion and extension films. There were no device-related adverse events.

In a separate study, 10 patients received TOPS implantation after total laminectomy and bilateral facetectomy for spinal stenosis at L3-L4 or L4-L5.[26,27] In two publications, outcomes were followed up for 11 years. Lasting improvements on VAS score for leg and back pain and ODI score were observed. There was no radiographic evidence of progression of spondylolisthesis in any of the cases, but one patient demonstrated asymptomatic stenosis adjacent to the index level. One patient experienced device failure in the form of a damaged and locked PcU component 12 weeks after implantation requiring conversion to instrumented fusion.

A phase 3 clinical trial, Safety and Effectiveness Study of the TOPS System, a Total Posterior Arthroplasty Implant Designed to Alleviate Pain Resulting From Moderate to Severe Lumbar Stenosis (NCT00405691), comparing TOPS to posterior spinal fusion with pedicle screws and local autograft bone after decompression for single-level moderate or severe spinal stenosis between L3 and L5 has been completed, and results have not yet been published. Currently, a new trial, A Pivotal Study of the Premia Spine TOPS System (NCT03012776), is ongoing. This trial seeks to assess whether TOPS is more effective than transforaminal lumbar interbody fusion when used to stabilize a single-level between L2 and L5 after decompression in patients with moderate-severe spinal stenosis, grade 1 spondylolisthesis or retrolisthesis, and thickening of the ligamentum flavum or scarring of the facet joint capsule.

Comparison

AFRS, TFAS, and TOPS were all studied in cadaveric models and demonstrated restoration of spinal biokinetics after decompression to near-physiologic levels. However, small differences in their designs led to various complications in clinical trials.

TFAS, which attaches to vertebral bodies using stems secured by bone cement, was shown to have durability issues in the form of stem breakage after implantation in two obese patients. This highlights the need to further study and optimize hardware durability preclinically with consideration of body habitus, which can place increased load on the device. Moreover, because the TFAS stems are secured with bone cement, posterior instrumented fusion was suboptimal as a salvage operation for these patients because of the risk of pseudoarthrosis. This secondary issue shows that future device design should allow for straightforward revision in the case of failure.

AFRS, being fully constructed from a metal alloy, induced cobalt allergies in 2 of 5 patients at a single institution, which required device removal and conversion to instrumented fusion. Because facet replacement devices are subjected to constant motion and stress throughout their indefinite lifespan, the release of immunogenic debris is an additional consideration beyond overall hardware durability.

TOPS addressed the aforementioned shortcomings of TFAS and AFRS with its design. Its PcU element captures debris while absorbing shock, which theoretically decreases the risk of construct failure. One reported case of device failure occurred 12 weeks after implantation and was due to a locked PcU component. The device design was subsequently revised to prevent future occurrence of this issue. Notably, for this patient, the screws used to secure the system were simply rotated and attached with rods to convert to instrumented fusion.[26]

With regard to clinical outcomes, all three devices have been shown in prospective studies to function appropriately as an alternative to instrumented fusion, with most patients reporting improvement of symptoms. While 4 of 13 patients receiving TFAS demonstrated radiographic progression of degeneration at the index and adjacent segments at a mean follow-up time of 3.7 years, this has not been observed in 29 patients receiving TOPS followed up to 1 year or in 10 patients followed up to 11 years. With regard to efficacy, the randomized clinical trial for TFAS was terminated early, and full results from AFRS and TOPS trials are currently unavailable. Preliminary results for AFRS suggest noninferiority to instrumented fusion. It thus remains to be seen whether facet replacement devices provide tangible benefit over instrumented fusion.

SUMMARY

Over the past two decades, there has been a push for the development of motion-preserving facet replacement devices as an alternative to rigid fixation and spinal fusion after decompressive laminectomy and facetectomy. The rationale for these devices stems from the hypothesis that by providing support while preserving the natural kinematics of the lumbar spine, they would simultaneously address pain associated with spinal instability, prevent development of instability after decompression surgery, and prevent abnormal load distribution associated with solid fusion,

which likely leads to adjacent segment degeneration/disease. While several devices have been developed, none to date have been proven to be more efficacious than rigid fixation and solid fusion after decompression for lumbar spinal stenosis. Among the devices discussed in the previous section, the TOPS holds the greatest promise, as patients receiving the device in its prospective nonrandomized trials have achieved durable symptomatic improvement lasting over a decade without progression of degeneration or significant hardware malfunction. Results of its randomized clinical trials remain to be seen.

CLINICS CARE POINTS

- Motion-preserving facet replacement devices, including AFRS, TFAS, and TOPS have been shown to preserve near-normal spinal motion while providing stability after laminectomy and bilateral facetectomy in ex vivo models.

- Clinical trials so far have demonstrated similar outcomes between facet arthroplasty and traditional fusion after decompression for lumbar spinal pathology.

- It remains to be seen whether facet arthroplasty improves clinical outcomes with regard to symptoms and the development of adjacent segment disease.

- A clinical trial for TOPS is ongoing and will provide additional information regarding the clinical utility of such devices.

REFERENCES

1. Ravindra VM, Senglaub SS, Rattani A, et al. Degenerative lumbar spine disease: estimating global incidence and worldwide volume. Global Spine J 2018; 8(8):784–94.
2. Chou R, Baisden J, Carragee EJ, et al. Surgery for low back pain: a review of the evidence for an american pain society clinical practice guideline. Spine 2009;34(10):1094–109.
3. Matsunaga S, Ijiri K, Hayashi K. Nonsurgically managed patients with degenerative spondylolisthesis: a 10-to 18-year follow-up study. J Neurosurg 2000;93(2):194–8.
4. Deyo RA, Gray DT, Kreuter W, et al. United states trends in lumbar fusion surgery for degenerative conditions. Spine 2005;30(12):1441–5.
5. Panjabi MM. Clinical spinal instability and low back pain. J Electromyogr Kinesiol 2003;13(4):371–9.

6. Pope MH, Panjabi M. Biomechanical definitions of spinal instability. Spine 1985;10(3):255–6.

7. Deyo RA, Nachemson A, Mirza SK. Spinal-fusion surgery—the case for restraint. Spine J 2004;4(5): S138–42.

8. Boos N, Webb JK. Pedicle screw fixation in spinal disorders: a European view. Eur Spine J 1997;6(1): 2–18.

9. Mulholland RC, Sengupta DK. Rationale, principles and experimental evaluation of the concept of soft stabilization, . Arthroplasty of the spine. Springer; 2004. p. 142–9.

10. Park P, Garton HJ, Gala VC, et al. Adjacent segment disease after lumbar or lumbosacral fusion: review of the literature. Spine 2004;29(17):1938–44.

11. Fischgrund JS, Mackay M, Herkowitz HN, et al. 1997 volvo award winner in clinical studies: Degenerative lumbar spondylolisthesis with spinal stenosis: a prospective, randomized study comparing decompressive laminectomy and arthrodesis with and without spinal instrumentation. Spine 1997;22(24): 2807–12.

12. Resnick DK, Choudhri TF, Dailey AT, et al. Guidelines for the performance of fusion procedures for degenerative disease of the lumbar spine. part 9: fusion in patients with stenosis and spondylolisthesis. J Neurosurg Spine 2005;2(6):679–85.

13. Carl A. Lumbar facet morphology and the development of an anatomic facet joint replacement (AFR), 6th annual meeting of the Spine Arthroplasty Society 2006. p. 9–13.

14. Rieker CB, Schön R, Köttig P. Development and validation of a second-generation metal-on-metal bearing: laboratory studies and analysis of retrievals. J Arthroplasty 2004;19(8):5–11.

15. Howie DW, McCalden RW, Nawana NS, et al. The long-term wear of retrieved McKee-farrar metal-on-metal total hip prostheses. J Arthroplasty 2005; 20(3):350–7.

16. Goel VK, Mehta A, Jangra J, et al. Anatomic facet replacement system (AFRS) restoration of lumbar segment mechanics to intact: a finite element study and in vitro cadaver investigation. SAS J 2007;1(1): 46–54.

17. Myer J, Youssef JA, Rahn KA, et al. ACADIA® facet replacement system IDE study: preliminary outcomes at two-and four-years postoperative. Spine J 2014;14(11):S160–1.

18. Goodwin ML, Spiker WR, Brodke DS, et al. Failure of facet replacement system with metal-on-metal bearing surface and subsequent discovery of cobalt allergy: report of 2 cases. J Neurosurg Spine 2018; 29(1):81–4.

19. Phillips FM, Tzermiadianos MN, Voronov LI, et al. Effect of the total facet arthroplasty system after complete laminectomy-facetectomy on the biomechanics of implanted and adjacent segments. Spine J 2009;9(1):96–102.

20. Zhu Q, Larson CR, Sjovold SG, et al. Biomechanical evaluation of the total facet arthroplasty system™: 3-dimensional kinematics. Spine 2007;32(1):55–62.

21. Voronov LI, Havey RM, Rosler DM, et al. L5–S1 segmental kinematics after facet arthroplasty. Int J Spine Surg 2009;3(2):50–8.

22. Sjovold SG, Zhu Q, Bowden A, et al. Biomechanical evaluation of the total facet arthroplasty system-®(TFAS®): Loading as compared to a rigid posterior instrumentation system. Eur Spine J 2012;21(8): 1660–73.

23. Vermesan D, Prejbeanu R, Daliborca CV, et al. A new device used in the restoration of kinematics after total facet arthroplasty. Med Devices (Auckl) 2014;7:157.

24. Palmer DK, Inceoglu S, Cheng WK. Stem fracture after total facet replacement in the lumbar spine: A report of two cases and review of the literature. Spine J 2011;11(7):e15–9.

25. McAfee P, Khoo LT, Pimenta L, et al. Treatment of lumbar spinal stenosis with a total posterior arthroplasty prosthesis: Implant description, surgical technique, and a prospective report on 29 patients. Neurosurg Focus 2007;22(1):1–11.

26. Anekstein Y, Floman Y, Smorgick Y, et al. Seven years follow-up for total lumbar facet joint replacement (TOPS) in the management of lumbar spinal stenosis and degenerative spondylolisthesis. Eur Spine J 2015;24(10):2306–14.

27. Smorgick Y, Mirovsky Y, Floman Y, et al. Long-term results for total lumbar facet joint replacement in the management of lumbar degenerative spondylolisthesis. J Neurosurg Spine 2019;32(1): 36–41.

Statement of Ownership, Management, and Circulation
POSTAL SERVICE® (All Periodicals Publications Except Requester Publications)

UNITED STATES POSTAL SERVICE®

1. Publication Title	2. Publication Number	3. Filing Date
NEUROSURGERY CLINICS OF NORTH AMERICA	010 – 548	9/18/2021

4. Issue Frequency	5. Number of Issues Published Annually	6. Annual Subscription Price
JAN, APR, JUL OCT	4	$438.00

7. Complete Mailing Address of Known Office of Publication *(Not printer) (Street, city, county, state, and ZIP+4®)*

ELSEVIER INC.
230 Park Avenue, Suite 800
New York, NY 10169

Contact Person
Malathi Samayan

Telephone *(Include area code)*
01-44-4299-4507

8. Complete Mailing Address of Headquarters or General Business Office of Publisher *(Not printer)*

ELSEVIER INC.
230 Park Avenue, Suite 800
New York, NY 10169

9. Full Names and Complete Mailing Addresses of Publisher, Editor, and Managing Editor *(Do not leave blank)*

Publisher *(Name and complete mailing address)*
DOLORES MELONI, ELSEVIER INC.
1600 JOHN F KENNEDY BLVD. SUITE 1800
PHILADELPHIA, PA 19103-2899

Editor *(Name and complete mailing address)*
STACY EASTMAN, ELSEVIER INC.
1600 JOHN F KENNEDY BLVD. SUITE 1800
PHILADELPHIA, PA 19103-2899

Managing Editor *(Name and complete mailing address)*
PATRICK MANLEY, ELSEVIER INC.
1600 JOHN F KENNEDY BLVD. SUITE 1800
PHILADELPHIA, PA 19103-2899

10. Owner *(Do not leave blank. If the publication is owned by a corporation, give the name and address of the corporation immediately followed by the names and addresses of all stockholders owning or holding 1 percent or more of the total amount of stock. If not owned by a corporation, give the names and addresses of the individual owners. If owned by a partnership or other unincorporated firm, give its name and address as well as those of each individual owner. If the publication is published by a nonprofit organization, give its name and address.)*

Full Name	Complete Mailing Address
WHOLLY OWNED SUBSIDIARY OF REED/ELSEVIER, US HOLDINGS	1600 JOHN F KENNEDY BLVD. SUITE 1800 PHILADELPHIA, PA 19103-2899

11. Known Bondholders, Mortgagees, and Other Security Holders Owning or Holding 1 Percent or More of Total Amount of Bonds, Mortgages, or Other Securities. If none, check box ▶ ☐ None

Full Name	Complete Mailing Address
N/A	

12. Tax Status *(For completion by nonprofit organizations authorized to mail at nonprofit rates) (Check one)*
The purpose, function, and nonprofit status of this organization and the exempt status for federal income tax purposes:
☒ Has Not Changed During Preceding 12 Months
☐ Has Changed During Preceding 12 Months *(Publisher must submit explanation of change with this statement)*

PS Form **3526**, July 2014 *[Page 1 of 4 (see instructions page 4)]* PSN: 7530-01-000-9931 **PRIVACY NOTICE:** See our privacy policy on www.usps.com

---

13. Publication Title	14. Issue Date for Circulation Data Below
NEUROSURGERY CLINICS OF NORTH AMERICA	JULY 2021

15. Extent and Nature of Circulation		Average No. Copies Each Issue During Preceding 12 Months	No. Copies of Single Issue Published Nearest to Filing Date
a. Total Number of Copies *(Net press run)*		132	121
b. Paid Circulation *(By Mail and Outside the Mail)*	(1) Mailed Outside-County Paid Subscriptions Stated on PS Form 3541 (Include paid distribution above nominal rate, advertiser's proof copies, and exchange copies)	52	44
	(2) Mailed In-County Paid Subscriptions Stated on PS Form 3541 (Include paid distribution above nominal rate, advertiser's proof copies, and exchange copies)	0	0
	(3) Paid Distribution Outside the Mails Including Sales Through Dealers and Carriers, Street Vendors, Counter Sales, and Other Paid Distribution Outside USPS®	47	45
	(4) Paid Distribution by Other Classes of Mail Through the USPS (e.g. First-Class Mail®)	0	0
c. Total Paid Distribution *(Sum of 15b (1), (2), (3), and (4))* ▶		99	89
d. Free or Nominal Rate Distribution *(By Mail and Outside the Mail)*	(1) Free or Nominal Rate Outside-County Copies included on PS Form 3541	17	14
	(2) Free or Nominal Rate In-County Copies Included on PS Form 3541	0	0
	(3) Free or Nominal Rate Copies Mailed at Other Classes Through the USPS (e.g. First-Class Mail)	0	0
	(4) Free or Nominal Rate Distribution Outside the Mail (Carriers or other means)	0	0
e. Total Free or Nominal Rate Distribution *(Sum of 15d (1), (2), (3) and (4))* ▶		17	14
f. Total Distribution *(Sum of 15c and 15e)* ▶		116	103
g. Copies not Distributed *(See instructions to Publishers #4 (page #3))* ▶		16	18
h. Total *(Sum of 15f and g)* ▶		132	121
i. Percent Paid *(15c divided by 15f times 100)* ▶		85.34%	86.4%

* If you are claiming electronic copies, go to line 16 on page 3. If you are not claiming electronic copies, skip to line 17 or page 3.

16. Electronic Copy Circulation		Average No. Copies Each Issue During Preceding 12 Months	No. Copies of Single Issue Published Nearest to Filing Date
a. Paid Electronic Copies ▶			
b. Total Paid Print Copies (Line 15c) + Paid Electronic Copies (Line 16a) ▶			
c. Total Print Distribution (Line 15f) + Paid Electronic Copies (Line 16a) ▶			
d. Percent Paid (Both Print & Electronic Copies) (16b divided by 16c × 100) ▶			

☐ I certify that 50% of all my distributed copies (electronic and print) are paid above a nominal price.

17. Publication of Statement of Ownership
☒ If the publication is a general publication, publication of this statement is required. Will be printed in the OCTOBER 2021 issue of this publication. ☐ Publication not required.

18. Signature and Title of Editor, Publisher, Business Manager, or Owner	Date
Malathi Samayan - Distribution Controller *Malathi Samayan*	9/18/2021

I certify that all information furnished on this form is true and complete. I understand that anyone who furnishes false or misleading information on this form or who omits material or information requested on the form may be subject to criminal sanctions (including fines and imprisonment) and/or civil sanctions (including civil penalties).

PS Form **3526**, July 2014 *(Page 3 of 4)* **PRIVACY NOTICE:** See our privacy policy on www.usps.com

Moving?

Make sure your subscription moves with you!

To notify us of your new address, find your **Clinics Account Number** (located on your mailing label above your name), and contact customer service at:

Email: journalscustomerservice-usa@elsevier.com

800-654-2452 (subscribers in the U.S. & Canada)
314-447-8871 (subscribers outside of the U.S. & Canada)

Fax number: 314-447-8029

Elsevier Health Sciences Division
Subscription Customer Service
3251 Riverport Lane
Maryland Heights, MO 63043

*To ensure uninterrupted delivery of your subscription, please notify us at least 4 weeks in advance of move.

ELSEVIER

Printed and bound by CPI Group (UK) Ltd, Croydon, CR0 4YY

08/05/2025

01864697-0012